What I Learned From Dad

WHAT I LEARNED FROM DAD

CARING FOR DAD THROUGH ALZHEIMER'S DISEASE

Honoring your Mother and Father can bring
some of God's greatest blessings!

CHUCK HORSTMAN

XULON PRESS

Xulon Press
555 Winderley Pl, Suite 225
Maitland, FL 32751
407.339.4217
www.xulonpress.com

© 2024 by Chuck Horstman

All rights reserved solely by the author. The author guarantees all contents are original and do not infringe upon the legal rights of any other person or work. No part of this book may be reproduced in any form without the permission of the author.

Due to the changing nature of the Internet, if there are any web addresses, links, or URLs included in this manuscript, these may have been altered and may no longer be accessible. The views and opinions shared in this book belong solely to the author and do not necessarily reflect those of the publisher. The publisher therefore disclaims responsibility for the views or opinions expressed within the work.

Unless otherwise indicated, Scripture quotations are from the EasyEnglish Bible Copyright © MissionAssist 2019 - Charitable Incorporated Organisation 1162807. Used by permission. All rights reserved.

Some names have been changed.

Paperback ISBN-13: 979-8-86850-247-7
Ebook ISBN-13: 979-8-86850-248-4

Table of Contents

Chapter 1   God Lets Us Know He Is in Control..............1

Chapter 2   Caring for Dad 7

Chapter 3   Our Struggles With Alzheimer's Disease...... 17

Chapter 4   Fall of 2021 27

Chapter 5   The Beginning of a Pivotal Year............... 39

Chapter 6   We Decide to Move 49

Chapter 7   Spring Break 55

Chapter 8   Life in the New House 67

Chapter 9   Beginning of the End........................... 71

Chapter 10   Preparations For a Tough Decision........... 81

Chapter 11   Second Surgery 89

Chapter 12   The Final Days 101

Chapter 13   Life After Dad 109

Bibliography 121

Prologue

OUR LIVES ARE lived out in chapters, so to speak. All of the chapters are intertwined and some have more significance than others. Our Loving Father is a master in assimilating the chapters into the "book" that is our life and all of the chapters are for our good. Nothing is ever brought or allowed into our lives unless God approves and it is part of His plan. This is demonstrated to us in the Holy Bible in the life of Job. In this story, we learn that even Satan has to receive permission from God to bring any harm to Job. Job's confident faith in God remains intact even when he doesn't understand why hardship is coming to him and his family. We all experience hardships throughout our lives and we have a choice as to how we will face these. These times will "make or break" us. I desire that this story of one of the most significant "chapters" of our lives, will encourage you that no matter how difficult circumstances become, God is always in control and He will bring good into your life as you obey and follow Him.

Let me begin by introducing who we are. I am the oldest of five children, three girls, Tina, Mishelle, and Charlotte, and two boys Gary and me. We were born to George and Sharon Horstman during the 1960s and 1970s. We had a two-parent home with a Christian Dad and Mom, who kept God and church a major part of our lives. I can't thank Dad and Mom enough for that!

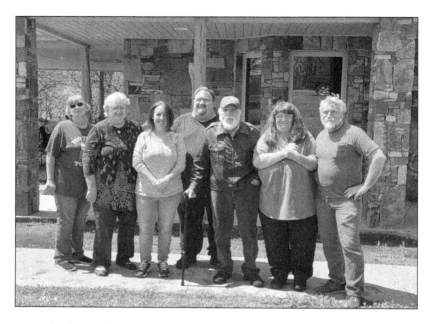

Chuck's Dad, Mon and Siblings in 2021. Chuck is in the blue shirt.

Julia and I married in 1988 after we met at Northeastern State University in Tahlequah, where we were both preparing to become teachers. She has been such a blessing in my life. Yes, we have had our ups and downs but I can always be assured that she is willing to meet me in the middle and we will stick it out through thick and thin. Overcoming the challenges has made us stronger and able to love more deeply than we did before we faced each challenge. More on that later.

Julia had two boys, Jeremy and Jason, from her first marriage and these boys have become my boys. I am so grateful for their willingness to allow me to be their dad and part of their family. I haven't been able to produce children, and I believe God had this plan for me to have a family. Jeremy and Jason both have married and we now have several grandchildren who have been a continued and expanded fulfillment of joy in my and Julia's lives. My family has been an enriching part of my life. There are many stories

Prologue

that I could share involving our boys and grand kids, but that isn't why I am writing this.

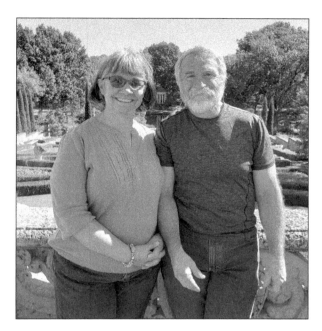

Chuck and wife, Julia in 2021

During her childhood, Julia and her family lived the majority of their lives as a family in the Tulsa area. During my childhood years, my family primarily lived in the Kiamichi Valley of southeastern Oklahoma in the small town of Muse.

After Julia and I completed our teaching degrees, our employment search led us to Alaska for five years. We taught the first year in a whaling village of around three hundred people and the following four years were in a larger village. Both of these villages are in the far northwest borough of Alaska. After those five years, we moved back to Oklahoma in 1995.

During the first summer back in Oklahoma in 1995, several events occurred that would shape our future: My parents divorced, Dad's oldest brother passed away, Julia's mom's brother passed away, and Julia's brother, Will, was arrested and sent to prison for several years. Will had been in and out of trouble with the law most of his life. During this incident, Julia's mom and dad, Joy and James, were in California as Joy's brother was passing away, they didn't need to deal with this also, so we did what we could concerning Will on this end in Oklahoma. It would have been difficult for us to return to Alaska after that summer after dealing with these issues. So God arranged things so we would be in Oklahoma instead.

Later, Will was released from prison and James and Joy did what they could to help him, but he never tried to stand on his own two feet. His parents continued to finance Will, so he never had to work for anything. Events involving Will during the next years set the stage for the story that I am sharing with you.

Eventually, around 2003, Joy started exhibiting symptoms of Alzheimer's disease and James asked us to help with caring for her. This led to us moving in with Julia's parents a few years later and my dad moving into our house. We bought the house when we moved back from Alaska in 1995. Little did we know that Dad later would also come down with Alzheimer's disease and would need us to get him through that stage of his life. We had intended to sell our house when we moved in with Julia's folks but God knew we would eventually need the house to care for Dad, so our efforts to sell the house failed. We were disappointed at the time that the house didn't sell, but in hindsight, we are now thankful that it didn't. God always knows what He is doing.

A few years later after Joy passed away in 2011, Julia and I moved back into our house with Dad to care for him. James remained in the house in which we had been living with him. Will was going to care for James while James lived there. The events that facilitated this move will be discussed in more detail later as those events had a major part of the story. I began recording the events of our lives when we moved into the house with Dad to care for him.

As Julia began helping James and Joy, one of the first issues they needed help with was their finances. It was revealed that Joy and Will had managed to get James and Joy several thousand dollars in debt. Most of this is due to all the money Joy had given to Will, mostly by borrowing it. James was angry at Will and didn't want to provide him with any more financial support. Throughout their lives, Joy handled Julia's parents' finances resulting in James not always being aware of everything that was happening. Joy's dementia played a part in this near the end, but James seemed to be kept from knowing how much money was going to her brother for several years. Julia spent several months getting their finances in order and dealing with the creditors and banks.

Also, years ago, Julia's parents bought a house for Will after he returned from prison for the first time so he had a place to live. Julia's parents wanted Julia to inherit the family house that they lived in when Julia and her brother were children. Julia's dad was upset at Will at the time and didn't want him to get the family house. So in 2005, Julia's parents signed the house over to Julia with the understanding that her parents could live in the house as long as they wanted. James and Joy took Julia to a notary public in Owasso to have the quit deed notarized. Julia took the deed to the recording office, putting the house in her name. We later moved the house into our trust.

Years later after Joy had passed away, Will began working his way back into good graces with James. Eventually, Will got it into James's head that Julia and I were stealing from James and mistreating him. One major piece of this story concerns the family home that Julia's parents had given to Julia. Will brainwashed James into thinking that we had tricked or cheated him and their mom out of the house, even though giving the house to Julia was

James's idea. Will claimed that we had been stealing from their parents. But we never took anything from them. Evidence verified that we hadn't.

It was during this time after Joy passed away in 2011 that my dad started exhibiting the symptoms of Alzheimer's disease and began needing help more and more. So we became torn between helping both of our dads. Moving Dad in with us where we lived with James wasn't prudent or in God's plan. But God will take care of that problem for us.

Hopefully, this provides you with an understanding of the setting and who is involved in our story.

Summer of 2018

In July of 2018, Julia and I took a two-week road trip to celebrate our 30th anniversary. When we returned from our anniversary trip, James started insisting that he wanted the house back in his name. Now he claiming that his original intent when signing the house over to Julia was for us to give the house back to him when he wanted it. He claimed that since he and Joy were in so much debt and bill collectors were calling, he was afraid that the creditors would be able to take the house from them to pay the bills and that was why he put the house in her name. But Julia had dealt with the creditors for them, so that wasn't a concern. However, we wouldn't sign the house back into Julia's dad's name as we were convinced that Will would then convince James to sell the house and give the money to him. Julia would never see the house again.

James continued to ask us off and on about signing the house over to him, but we always refused. When signing the house to Julia, James had stated specifically that he and Joy wanted Julia to have the house since they had given so much to Will as well as a house throughout the years. Yes, Julia's parents had helped Julia through some tough times also as parents do, but Julia's brother had exploited his parents all of his life.

Prologue

Eventually, with Will's prompting and design, in late October of that year, Julia's dad went to the courthouse to file for a restraining order and eviction against us, successfully getting us put out of the house that was legally ours. He also sued us attempting to get the house back in his name and payment for damages for allegedly stealing from him. This action by James was used by God to let us know that we were now free to help Dad. Will, we assumed would help their dad. James obviously didn't want us to be with him. So we didn't continue to feel an obligation to care for James as we had before. We believe Will was hoping to serve the eviction and lawsuit to us on Julia's birthday on October 13th, but the eviction and notice didn't happen until October 18th.

Between the time we returned from our anniversary trip and the eviction, we spent most of our time with Dad as he needed more care. Each evening we would return to the house with James after Dad was fed and ready for bed. At this point, Dad was able to sleep through the night alone. Each morning we would return to the house with Dad or I would go to teach school and Julia would go stay with Dad. I would go to Dad's house after school for dinner.

At this point any time we spent with James, he was not pleasant and at times ugly to us. This was discouraging to Julia and she didn't enjoy spending time with her dad like she had. Her dad was becoming more critical and demeaning to her. So she preferred to be at Dad's anyway. She would be sure to come home to fix dinner for James but often he wouldn't eat what she fixed and would fix his own meals. So we had been eating dinner with Dad and only going back to the house to sleep. So moving in with Dad was a natural transition for us.

The pivotal morning was a Sunday morning on October 18th as we were preparing to go to church, when the sheriff's deputy showed up, with Will in the lead, to serve the eviction and lawsuit notice. As painful as this was, it turned out to be a hugely positive change for us. When the eviction notice was served to us, we had an hour to get as many of our things as we could removed from the house. The van and car were packed full before we left a little over an hour later. After our first and only court hearing, we were able to get more from the house. The judge ruled that her dad had no right to keep us out of the house and he didn't have the right to put us out in the first place. The judge also noted that she could see no grounds for any of their claims against us. Will had come to the courthouse in a suit and tie with a smug look on his face. That all changed when the judge ruled against them. In fact, Will had to leave the courtroom before the hearing as he was a potential witness and our lawyer asked that Will and his wife as potential witnesses, be sequestered. James and Will pursued the lawsuit anyway.

We submitted all for which we were subpoenaed for the lawsuit as required. During the discovery process of the court proceedings, Will and James were in for disappointment as there was no evidence that we had stolen anything because we hadn't. Also, it was obvious that the house belonged to us. But we had promised that James could stay in the house as long as he wanted, so we never told him that he needed to leave the house. That would have to be his choice.

In addition to the lawsuit, James and Will reported to the Adult Protective Services that we were abusing James, which wasn't true. Those claims were rejected by the Adult Protective Services as false. Neither were any financial abuse or theft found during their investigation. But Adult Protective Services said that James could pursue damages in civil court if he so desired. Hence the lawsuit. We eventually settled out of court with James in November of 2021 without ever going back to court.

At the time of the eviction, we moved in with Dad not realizing at the time that God was using James and Will's actions to accomplish His will in our lives in major ways other than freeing us to care for Dad. One huge event

Prologue

for me came later on the day of the eviction. As I was praying God spoke to me in a clear voice, "I want you!" I just broke down in tears for a while. As much as the day's actions hurt, God was working things for our good. As I stated earlier, before this happened we had been torn knowing that Dad needed more and more help but we had committed to helping Julia's dad. Now we understood that our place was with Dad. James was now relying on Will to help him with what he needed.

There was one other time during this ordeal when God spoke so clearly to me. During fall break the following year in 2019, I asked if any of my siblings would be willing to come sit with Dad so Julia and I could get away even for one night. But all of them said that they had plans and wouldn't be able to help. So I was discouraged and was basically pouting. As I sat pouting about how unfair this was, God spoke again to me saying, "Quit trying to mess up what I want to do for you!" Again, confirming that He was with us through all of this and in control of all things. God is always good, no matter our circumstances.

Both of these incidents have increased my sensitivity to God's voice. I will never forget these times as this was God's way of meeting my needs specifically. Even if He never speaks to me this way again, I pray that I will be in tune with God so that I don't miss anything that He wants me to hear. And if he wants to reassure me audibly, I don't want to miss that either.

It was when we moved in with Dad after the eviction that I began keeping a journal of the events of our lives during our time with Dad. That journal is the primary material for this book. I originally began keeping a record because I had an understanding that God intended for me to share at Dad's funeral. I had no way of knowing if I would be able to pull off speaking at Dad's funeral service. God provided more confirmation for me in different ways that, "Yes", I was to speak at Dad's service.

The first of these confirmations occurred during spring break of 2022 in March. This is one of the two times we used respite care for Dad. Respite care was being provided by LifePace, an organization only 15 miles away in Tulsa that provided support for Julia and me in caring for Dad. During this week of spring break, Dad's sister, Aunt Carolyn passed away. Since Dad was being cared for and I was out of school for the week, we were able to attend her funeral service.

After the funeral service at the church, Charlotte rode with Julia and me to Aunt Carolyn's graveside service and a discussion of Dad's impending service arose. Charlotte asked who I thought should preach at Dad's service. For the first time, I admitted that I felt that I was supposed to be the one. Charlotte was surprised and asked if I was sure I could do that. I admitted that I didn't know how, but if God intended for me to do then He would provide what I needed. Then she said that she felt like she was to sing at his service and had the same angst that I had. As it turned out, in the end, we both fulfilled what we had discussed on that day because we felt that God called us to do it. God provided what we needed to go through something so difficult.

Another major confirmation was a note I found written by Dad in 2006 years before. I had asked Dad to record what he would like to have as part of his final service in a booklet that I had received from a funeral home. I had him do this before any symptoms of Alzheimer's disease were present. We knew the day would come and I wanted him to let us know his wishes while he was able. I put the book away and didn't look at it until after he passed away. In the last section of the booklet, he wrote that as a part of his service "I would like my kids to say something." This brought me to tears knowing that God is working things out all along even years before I had any notion of what would transpire.

I will never regret being obedient to God's direction when His desires are so obvious. Being obedient isn't always easy though. The seventh commandment from Exodus 20:12 states, "Always respect your father and your mother. Then you will live for many years in the land that the Lord your God will give to you." something Julia and I tried to do as best we could.

Jesus taught more on this subject in Matthew 15:4, 5, and 6 when rebuking the religious leaders:

> [4] *God's Law says: "You must love your father and mother and obey them." God also said, "A person should die if he says bad things against his father or against his mother."* [5] *But you teach that a person may say to his father or to his mother, "I would have given gifts to help you. But I cannot do that because I have given them to God instead."* [6] *Then, you let that person give nothing to his parents. He does not have to help them. This shows that you have not obeyed what God says is right. Instead, you have obeyed your own ideas.*

I believe it is God's desire for us to care for our parents to honor them. My prayer is that from this story, you will be encouraged to be obedient to God even if the path before you appears to be difficult or even impossible, as ours seemed to be at times. But when you are in God's will, God provides you with what you need.

Chapter 1

God Lets Us Know He Is in Control

As KIDS, WE spent time on family trips and vacations. There were times when Dad would work away from home, and Mom kept the home fires burning. All five of us children have good memories of our childhood. Of course, with all families, we had our difficulties and challenges. We tend to want to forget those times, but God has given me a different perspective on how to view these experiences.

Throughout my life, God let me know that He is in control in various ways. We don't have control over who are parents will be, so I am thankful to have Christian parents. I have to give God credit for this. We could count on going to church. Again, no church (or any organization staffed with fallible humans) isn't without flaws. But as with my home life, I have many fond memories of my church life. Primarily, I cherish the Word of God that I learned all those years. Many times Julia would ask me a question about something in the Bible and I would know the answer due to something that I learned in Sunday school, VBS, or during a sermon that I heard while a young person. One of my primary regrets is that I didn't always take what I learned and apply it to my life as consistently as I should have. I have a Biblical understanding of life from my childhood upbringing.

Even after Mom and Dad divorced, they would both join us at family events as our parents for holidays, birthdays, and other special events. I have always appreciated that, as togetherness doesn't always happen in families with divorce. On the day that we were preparing to enter the chapel for Dad's funeral, it crossed my mind that even divorce can't break a family circle that God has put together. We have a wonderful God!

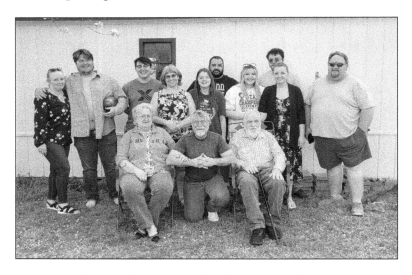

Chuck, Julia, Mom, Dad and Gary with Chuck & Julia's son, Jason and his family in 2019.

Another thing is I have always loved kids and enjoy being with them. I anticipated one day having a daughter of my own. That never happened. But when I was thirteen, Mom had Charlotte. Charlotte and I became best buddies and had great times. We have been close, and enjoyed life together, especially our childhood. We continue to have a special bond. I also have granddaughters who are a source of joy. God has always provided special relationships that have enriched my life.

There were the events that led me to meet Julia. It all began when I asked to be assigned to a specific school for my elementary internship. But I received my assignment, it was at a different school. When I asked my advisor what caused the change she said she made a mistake calling the wrong school. Even though I said that I was willing to stay where I was, at

God Lets Us Know He Is in Control

her insistence, she was able to get me reassigned to the school that I had requested. I met Julia at that school. We may never have met if I had stayed with the first school.

There have been too many of these circumstances in my life to call them coincidence.

Another major example of God's intervention in our lives occurred while we were in Alaska. Julia and I both taught school there from 1990 to 1995. In one situation many specific and timely pieces had to fit together. God organized many of those events so that they fit together perfectly in 24 hours.

We had started in a small whaling village, Kivalina. During the year, we felt that we needed to move into a larger village the next school year. In the spring we applied for positions in Kotzebue, a larger village for the upcoming school year not knowing for sure that we would be accepted for teaching positions there. As our first year in Kivalina was coming to an end, we made preparations to move to Kotzebue.

To add to the uncertainty of what we would be doing the following school year, there were some unusual events through which God clearly revealed His unique way of working through events in our lives. First of all, there was a fire in the phone interchange in Kotzebue and all communication from the area of Kotzebue and the surrounding villages, including ours, was cut off. There was no way for any communication between villages, towns, or the rest of the world. We couldn't even communicate with the airlines to ensure that we would be able to get out of Kivalina to Kotzebue and beyond as we were going home for the summer. We had made reservations, but we couldn't confirm our flights the day before the flight was expected.

But the plane was on time and we got to Kotzebue on a Thursday evening after we had finished all our obligations at Kivalina. On Friday morning, we went to the school offices in Kotzebue to talk to the school officials who

What I Learned From Dad

told us that a meeting was scheduled at 1:00 that afternoon to fill open positions in the school in Kotzebue and we were in consideration for positions. So we waited to hear if we would have teaching positions in Kotzebue for the following school year.

Meanwhile, as we waited, we learned that one phone line had been reestablished, finally allowing communication outside of Kotzebue. The elementary school was open and we were allowed to look around the school. While there, Julia encountered a teacher who was clearing out the last of her things from the school as she and her husband were going back home to Arkansas. During the conversation, the teacher who was leaving mentioned that the house they had been renting was available. She gave Julia the contact information for the owners of the house who lived in Anchorage.

Another piece of the puzzle was our belongings were sitting in the Kotzebue post office, around twenty-five boxes, that we shipped from Kivalina. If we didn't get teaching positions in Kotzebue, we would need to go to the post office, relabel our boxes, and have them send them on to Oklahoma. Our flight to Oklahoma was leaving on Saturday morning with a four-hour layover in Anchorage.

Well as it turned out, later in the afternoon we were informed that both Julia and I were approved to be assigned to teaching positions in Kotzebue Elementary; Julia would teach first grade and I would teach fifth grade.

Here is where the timing became tight. I got in line to use the phone to call the owners of the house that was available for rent as we hoped to be able to rent the house. I don't remember how long I waited in line, but I was able to make contact with the owners. The owner said we could rent the house on the condition that we come to Anchorage to sign a contract, and pay the deposit and first month's rent, upfront. Well, it just happened that we had that four-hour layover at the Anchorage airport on our way through to Oklahoma. Just enough time to rent a car, drive to meet the owner, sign the contract, make the necessary payments, get back to the airport, and board the plane to continue our trip to Oklahoma. Our flight is scheduled to leave on Saturday morning and it is now Friday afternoon. It still amazes me the way God arranges things for us without our knowledge! We had purchased the plane tickets in January long before knowing how events would transpire at the end of the year. But God know all along when we needed to leave and that we needed that layover!!

There was one task left and we had just enough time to address it. That was the issue of our boxes in the post office in Kotzebue. After establishing that we could rent the house through the summer and the next school year, the owner said that we could get the keys from the teachers who were leaving. We had enough time to retrieve the boxes from the post office and place them in the house. That way our things would be there for us when we returned for the beginning of the next school year.

For the next four years, starting in 1991, we taught school together in Kotzebue. It wasn't long before God's desires for our lives in Kotzebue began to emerge. Even though we were in Kotzebue to teach school, God had us there to serve the local Assembly of God church. During the four years, I taught the adult Sunday School class and even spoke on Sunday mornings a couple of times when the pastor was out of town. Julia helped with the children and the women's ministry. I also played guitar for worship but never was able to play as well as I would have liked. We have great memories of our time in Alaska.

When our sons were getting into high school we moved back to Oklahoma in 1995. We especially relish the memories of how God was at work in our lives. And God isn't done.

After settling in Oklahoma in 1995, Julia and I bought a house and taught in different public schools in Oklahoma. Julia was teaching in the same school her mom had spent teaching for the majority of her career.

After teaching four years I took a position as an administrator at a private Christian school until 2008. Years later after Jeremy and Jason were grown and starting their own families, grand kids were our new passion and life was good and progressing as expected.

However, a few years after Julia's mom, Joy retired, and began having difficulty with her cognitive functioning and Julia's dad started needing help to care for her. This was around 2003. God arranged things, especially our finances to allow Julia to help with Joy. Julia began part-time work instead of full-time to have more time to help her parents. In time, Julia stopped working even part-time as Joy's needs required more extensive help. Joy was later diagnosed with Alzheimer's disease.

As Joy's needs increased, in 2006, we moved into the upstairs of James and Joy's house to be available at any time. I even resigned from administrative work at Rejoice Christian School in 2008 and took a teaching job in another town about 30 minutes away that would allow me to have more time available if needed, especially in the summers. Even with all of these life changes and reductions in financial income, we didn't always have a lot of discretionary cash, but we always had what we needed.

When we moved in with Julia's parents in 2006, we tried to sell our house in town, but that didn't happen. Since it didn't sell, my dad moved into our house as he was renting a small apartment and this would provide him more space and he would be closer to us. None of us had a clue that this house would be his final home on earth as he would also suffer from Alzheimer's disease. Also, in 2018, when Dad's needs required 24-hour care and the timing was right God arranged events so we would again be back in that house with Dad to provide that care.

Chapter 2

Caring for Dad

BETWEEN 2015 AND 2018, Dad started showing signs that he was declining. For example, Dad had cataract surgery and my brother Gary stayed with Dad to help him. Gary being with Dad those 4 or 5 days, illustrated the degree of decline to which Dad had slipped. Eventually, Julia and I would be there every day as Dad needed help with many day-to-day tasks such as shopping, cooking, cleaning, taking his medicine, finances, etc. Driving was becoming a concern, but thankfully Dad gave this up willingly.

I would put his medicine in a dispenser for the week so he could take it at the required times. One Monday, he took a week's worth of his medications at once requiring a night in the hospital for observation. His medications were locked away after that and given to him one dose at a time. This required more supervision and this need would increase to the point that either Julia or I needed to be there most of the day.

In 2018, I started my journal about caring for Dad. The reason I started this journal was so I could share it at Dad's funeral service. I knew this would not be a typical sermon, eulogy, speech, or whatever you want to call it that you hear at a memorial service or funeral. I don't know that this would be so much a memorial to Dad's life but more about the lessons God taught me through life with Dad. The last years starting around 2015, of caring for Dad were used by God to bring me closer to God than I have ever been. I have learned how to be a better husband to Julia, who is one of the greatest blessings that God has given me in this life. She is such an angel, especially in caring for others. I wouldn't give anything for the time we had together, especially in the time of caring for Dad, and Joy, as both were going through the stages of Alzheimer's disease.

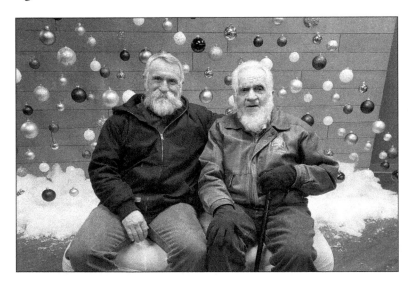

Chuck with Dad at Christmas in 2020.

I liked to describe Dad as a "throwback to the hippies". He wasn't a hippie but a lot of his ways were reflective of the life view of the hippies, especially living more for the moment and taking care of what needed to be dealt with at that time. Many of his phrases were unique. One example, he needed to straighten out a bent metal fence post, which he did. Later on, one of our cousins, asked him how he got the post straight. He stated that he "put it in the crotch of a tree and commenced to prizing on it." Also, whenever as children we were energetic and began to get noisy in the house, he would tell us to go outside and run around the house "sixteen times". I never knew where the number "sixteen" came from and I don't know if he ever did either.

Caring for Dad

It wasn't always easy being a full-time caregiver for Dad. Watching other couples the same age as Julia and I have free time and finances to do many things we would have enjoyed provoked envy. It took a couple of times for God to press home the point to me that serving Dad was our assignment at this time. We appreciated Mom and my siblings giving us breaks now and then. But as Dad's needs increased those breaks became difficult as my siblings didn't always understand as well as Julia and I what Dad needs. I know Dad didn't choose or want the situation he endured but God had things prepared for his care. I remember becoming frustrated because Dad couldn't do something and Dad sensed my frustration. This resulted in him reacting angrily. I resolved to not get frustrated again as I had the ability to do so, with God's help, but Dad couldn't help getting angry due to his dementia.

Anyway, back to Dad's care as our assignment. I am learning what God meant when He said, "My thoughts are not like yours. Your ways are not like mine." Isaiah 55 verse 8. We prayed that Dad would continue to have an agreeable attitude and be easy to care for. He was for the most part. Julia was his primary caregiver as I continued to teach school, which was a 30-minute drive for me each day. Dad needed to allow Julia to help him for this arrangement to continue.

A few months after we moved in with Dad, he started having difficulty sleeping and would get up to wander the house. One night I caught him trying to go out the front door in his pajamas in the middle of the night. We acquired some door sensors that would alert us when the door was being opened. Then one night Dad fell while wandering around in his room, we added a motion sensor to wake me when he got out of bed. Some nights he would get up four or five times a night. After a few months, just when this became almost too much to bear, Dad started sleeping most of the night getting up once or twice, which was bearable.

Around this time I was led to Ann Voskamp's book "One Thousand Gifts"[1]. From her book, I learned more about the wisdom of unanswered prayers. I learned the power of gratitude and how gratitude leads to God's heart and blessings otherwise beyond our reach. For example, Jesus endured the agony of the cross because He was aware of the joy He would experience in the salvation his death and resurrection would provide us.

The kingdom of God is on earth. We can be a part of His kingdom if we submit our will to Him. I was reminded how important it is to realize that our lives are not our own. Some are here to bless and some are here to be blessed. Just as the Jews and the disciples had misunderstood Jesus' life on earth as one of servant hood, we misunderstand that the pursuit of earthly goals is futile. If we want to reap heavenly rewards, we have to surrender our lives to His desires. But this pursuit of heavenly goals and treasure is foolishness to the world. This only makes sense with the Holy Spirit in our lives.

When the COVID-19 pandemic hit in 2020, I prayed hard about God protecting us, especially Dad, from the Covid virus. So it was quite a blow when Julia then I started to exhibit symptoms. When Dad also contracted the illness, I was devastated. I was convinced that God would not let Dad catch Covid. But again God had other plans for us.

I had one night of chills, sweat, and light fever, on Wednesday, that was all. Combining that with Julia's headaches and other aches, all three of us were scheduled to take the COVID test on Friday morning. After submitting the samples that morning, Dad coughed all that night, just a light persistent cough. Saturday, he slept all day in his recliner with intermittent coughing and a low-grade fever below 100. His insurance company had sent a pulse oximeter, blood pressure cuff, and thermometer, so we watched his vitals and kept his doctor informed. His blood oxygen lingered in the 90s

---

[1] Voskamp, Ann, *One Thousand Gifts: A Dare to Live Fully Right Where You Are.* Grand Rapids, Mich., Zondervan, 2010. ISBN 9780310321910

with a couple of readings in the 80s. Then I read that cold skin will produce a low reading, and Dad often has cold hands, so from then on I warmed his finger by holding it in my hand before applying the oximeter. From then on Dad's oxygen levels stayed in the 90s.

Dad's blood pressure was never high and he didn't wheeze much when breathing. We received news of positive results on our Covid test on Sunday morning. For the most part, we seemed to be on the mend. We rested and continued to monitor Dad's oxygen levels and temperature. On Monday, I informed Dad's doctor of the positive test and sent him the vitals that I had logged over the weekend. His doctor asked if I would like to schedule Dad to have an infusion of monoclonal antibodies. After discussing it with my siblings, we said sure. So on Tuesday, I took Dad for the infusion. Dad handled it well.

Dad was dazed the rest of the day. Julia's symptoms hung on, especially the headaches. I was reading a book titled "Hope in the Dark"[2] by Craig Groeschel, pastor of Life Church. A good friend had given us the book as a gift. The author reminded us of the time Paul asked to have a thorn of flesh removed. But God told him that His Grace is sufficient. Paul seemed to need something in his life that required him to depend on God. Something we all need. It is hard for me to see Julia suffer and not be able to "fix" things for her or anyone else for that matter. This is hard for me as I have most of my life been able to fix most things on which I set my mind. I realize these are abilities and desires that God has given me and not of my own doing. God is still trying to keep me in my place, depending on Him, instead of my abilities. Don't get me wrong, He expects me to do what I can with the abilities that He gave me, but not to rely on myself and my abilities instead

---

[2] Groeschel, Craig, *Hope in the Dark,* Zondervan. 08/21/2018. ISBN-13: 9780310342953

of Him. A lesson long in learning for me. I also have to keep in mind that any ability I have comes from God.

As I stated, it was difficult for me when Dad first became ill with COVID-19 symptoms, I was devastated as I believed God would protect Dad from the disease since I had prayed that God would. But God didn't. So I leaned on my family, and siblings to pray as I was struggling. Dad came through on Saturday and Sunday fine. He slept and was disoriented but never struggled to breathe. God impressed me that I needed not fear the virus and that Dad was going to be fine. God wanted me to see that the threat of the virus was much worse than the actual infection. God was taking care of Dad through it and also teaching me to rely on Him through the ordeal. It then seemed to me that Dad was here at this time for me and Julia to teach us to rely on God and bring us into a closer relationship with Him.

I believe the last few years also helped Dad work through some issues in his life. Now Dad looks forward to Heaven more than ever. God is in the business of redemption to restore us to our relationship with Him!!! That is why Jesus suffered, to make this redemption possible for us. As with almost everyone else, Covid changed our lives for the next couple of years.

After about ten days of Covid effects, we all started to bounce back. I was reading through "One Thousand Gifts"[3] again and was impressed to reflect on the chapter when Ann's son's hand was damaged in a fan. He required surgery to repair his hand. When she returned home from the emergency room with her son she relayed to her Mother-in-law what had happened. After hearing the story, her Mother-in-law responded, "Well at least he still has his hand". It crossed Ann's mind, "So if my son had lost his hand, is God then not good?" The answer, of course, is "God is always good". In contrast to Ann's story, at the time this is happening with Ann's son, one of Ann's

---

[3] Voskamp, Ann, *One Thousand Gifts: A Dare to Live Fully Right Where You Are.* Grand Rapids, Mich., Zondervan, 2010. ISBN 9780310321910

neighbors was burying their son. Ann was impressed by the faith of the boy's family as the family thanked God for having the time they had with their son and still trusted God through the pain of losing him. The lesson to learn from the dilemma is that God is good all the time. The trick is to take time to let God show your life to you from His perspective, to put on the "glasses" that He gives us to see the good in everything.

I also returned to the book "Hope in the Dark"[4]. This book is based on the Biblical book of Habakkuk. Habakkuk was given a message from God that He was preparing the Babylonians, a vicious and evil nation, to punish Israel for their sinful ways. Habakkuk had been pleading out to God concerning Israel's wayward ways and asked how could God continue to ignore and tolerate Israel's evil. God told him that He was preparing a way to punish the Israelites and that Habakkuk would be shocked at what God would do to punish the Israelites. God is going to use the Babylonians, an evil people to punish Israel.

After working through his angst at the horrible Babylonians being used by God, Habakkuk praised God for His goodness and love for Israel and us. God always knows what is best. When we suffer the consequences of our sins, God's goodness allows those consequences to happen. When God destroyed Sodom and Gomorrah thereby punishing their sin, He was being just. God knows it isn't justice for those who do their best to shun evil if those who commit evil deeds aren't punished.

Even "bad" can happen to good people because God has better for them and will use everything for good to those who are called according to His purposes as stated by Paul in the book of Romans 8:28. So events that we label as "bad" don't qualify as such from God's perspective. Job is the prime example of this as he suffered much, and he didn't commit evil deeds to

---

[4] Groeschel, Craig, *Hope in the Dark*, Zondervan. 08/21/2018. ISBN-13: 9780310342953

bring the consequences he suffered. At the end of the book of Job, Job had a much better relationship and understanding of God from his experience.

Abraham made some mistakes and suffered consequences. However, the effects of those consequences increased his strength to the point that he was able to offer Isaac as a sacrifice. Isaac was the son God had given Abraham and Sarah to fulfill His promise to provide them with a son. Abraham and Sarah were both over 90 years old when Isaac was born to them, while Sarah was well past child bearing years. Isaac's birth was a miracle provided by God! This was the most difficult test of Abraham's life!! At the last minute, God provided a ram for the sacrifice just as Abraham raised the knife to slay Isaac. Even after waiting so long for Isaac, Abraham was convinced that God would keep His promise through Isaac, even if God had to raise Isaac from death.

Even the results of the fallen state in which we find ourselves, "bad" can happen to us with nobody at fault or committing sin. There is a great example of this in the Bible with the blind man healed by Jesus in the book of John chapter 9. When asked by Jesus who sinned and caused this man to be blind, Jesus said, "No one, not him or his parents." Instead, this man's present state was going to be an opportunity for God to be glorified. The end of the story has the man agreeing to become a follower of Jesus. To me, the point is, that it was beneficial to be blind part of his life and then find Jesus than for him to have had his vision all of his life and never find Jesus. Sounds harsh, well how harsh will eternity in hell be? Again, from whose perspective are you viewing life's circumstances?

God often uses the circumstances of others to work His will in our lives. If we are willing to be obedient and submissive to be a servant to others, we place ourselves in a position to reap heavenly rewards. The choice is up to us. Dad would want you to know that he is now in the arms of Jesus. He didn't ask to suffer dementia from Alzheimer's disease with its slow degrading of his life and dignity. But God arranged circumstances in preparation for this stage of his life and He also aligned Julia and my lives to meet Dad's needs and provide growth for Julia and me. Some of the best years of our marriage were during this time. We both grew closer to God during this time. So what may have looked to the world to be an unfortunate time had good for us. Following are some of the specifics of caring for Dad, especially the last year.

Don't get me wrong, most of the time, it wasn't that difficult caring for Dad. Much of what Dad needed at first was the equivalent of caring for a child. But as the disease progressed, his needs were more demanding. This was when I started making more detailed entries in my journal. Writing things down was very helpful for me in this journey. My prayer is that you will be encouraged to allow God to work His will in your life from our experiences.

Chapter 3

Our Struggles With Alzheimer's Disease

MARCH, 2021

OFTEN DAD HAS difficulty staying asleep at night, often waking and thinking that it is time to get up and do things. We can't let him wander the house on his own while we sleep as we don't know if he will wander outside or fall in the house. One night in particular, he was up over five times and I only got about three hours of sleep. I became upset at Dad which didn't help. I didn't get to sleep until it was 3:00 am. So I prayed beside his bed with him for quite a while. The doctor said to try to keep him as active as you can during the day to tire him, which we tried, but it seems nothing stops the effects of the dementia.

If Dad had a night when he was up often, I would turn off the sound of the motion sensor so that Julia would not also have to continue to be woken each time Dad got up. I would get up to wait for Dad to get sleepy again. If he wanted to come out of his room then I have to get up with him. Most of the time, I could get him talking a bit, then divert him back to bed or his room. If he wouldn't get back in bed, I would go sit in the other room listening as Dad would mosey around his room for a while, eventually, he would lay back down, often sideways, on the bed. After things became quiet, I realized that he was asleep, I would then get him back under the covers.

Julia and I kept praying for discernment and wisdom to handle the nuances of his dementia. Throughout my life, I've had a problem with waking up at night and worrying about things. God impressed me the next day that He wanted to help me with this through Dad. As long as my physical body can handle it..... I asked the siblings to pray that Dad sleeps better.

At this point I was led to Jennie Allen's book, "Get Out of Your Head"[5]. She wrote the book to address the need we have to protect our minds from the influences of the world and our enemy the devil. One of my major struggles was worrying about things, as I stated above. Daily life presents enough negative input to take in, and demonic forces will attack us with thoughts to bring doubts in our minds against God.

This was the method used with Eve. Through the serpent the devil put thoughts in her mind to produce doubt about God. Jennie wrote in her book that she suffered such attacks. I suspect that I have suffered similar attacks at points in my life when I had a hard time shaking certain negative thoughts often for extended times. These thoughts or worries would often keep me awake for hours. I started putting more priority on reading God's Word, listening to and watching God honoring content and music while avoiding anything contrary to God's Word. I did this, especially at bedtime. Julia and I made a more concentrated effort to spend time in devotions and prayer together. Reading about Jennie's experiences and her advice in her book was very helpful. At this point, It is very seldom that I have trouble sleeping due to negative thoughts or what I call "stinking thinking", a phrase I heard as a kid. I still listen to many of Jennie Allen's podcasts[6].

---

[5] Allen, Jennie, *Get Out of Your Head: Stopping the Spiral of Toxic Thoughts.* Crown Publishing Group, 2020. ISBN 9781601429667

[6] HTTP://www.jennieallen.com/podcast

August, 2021

I went to lunch with some of the teachers who I had worked with in the last few years. All of us will be working in different places beginning this year. Julia stayed with Dad at home so I could go. While I was there Dad had an accident and he wouldn't let Julia get him clean. So I hurried and finished lunch to get home. He allowed me to clean him when I got home but we knew that we were going to need some help soon.

So we started seeking avenues of support for us. The constant presence of dealing with Dad's needs was getting exhausting. It seemed earlier in the year when I searched for places, I kept hitting dead ends and we gave up. But this time my first inquiry was promising. I believe that we hadn't achieved all that God had in mind for us until this time, or both of us needed to learn something or grow in some way and until God was able to get us to the place He wanted us, so change wasn't going to happen. So it wasn't in God's will until now for us to have help with Dad.

Since I had been home for the summer as most school teachers, both of us had been available during the day, but now that school was starting again, Julia was left to burden the load by herself during the days. So before things became too difficult, we wanted to have something in place. One of the options that looked to be available included adult daycare, which would provide Dad with more interaction with others, something he seemed to enjoy. He will be able to receive some of his health care there, showers, some laundry services, and some time for Julia to be able to do more for herself. LifePace, the service we were seeking to use would become Dad's total care mechanism. We just had to get through the Medicaid Advantage application process, which can take six to eight weeks. We had four different interviews or sessions to complete the various applications that are part of the process. We were hopeful that services would begin on October 1st.

One note I want to make concerning one of the inquiries I made while searching for long-term care for Dad. I called Dad's primary care doctor for advice. The doctor had the social services branch of Utica Park Clinic call us. The counselor didn't take long to ask if I wanted to know how to get Dad into a nursing home. I told her that we desired assistance so we could keep him at home with us. Her tone becomes more excited and upbeat. She sounded as if she couldn't believe that was what we wanted. I assume that most of the time what she does in situations like ours is assist families with finding nursing home care. I explained that we were applying through LifePace and she said that sounded like what a great option. The way she acted what I said made her day.

It is heartbreaking to me that so many families take the easy way out. One of the other agents who assisted us in the application process said it is surprising the number of families who will put an aging family member in a nursing home and never look back. Now if Dad's needs eventually required residential care, I was not against that. But I won't neglect to see him and do all that I can for him. I knew that near the end of his life, this may be required. And I was becoming OK with that.

One other service provided by LifePace is respite care, in which Dad could be housed in a memory care facility for a short time so we could get some rest. This also allowed us to ease into Dad being in residential care if that were ever required. Julia and I were determined that as long as we were able, Dad would be at home with us.

Throughout the application process, other methods of support were emerging, but we felt that LifePace was the best option for us. We continued to pray for guidance. Also, the application process for LifePace would lay the groundwork for services from other sources, including hospice services that could begin in the later stages of his Alzheimer's disease with fewer services earlier on. More on that to come...

October 1, 2021

We have completed the Life Pace application process and Dad had his first day at the Adult Day Health Center (ADHC). We were able to tour the north facility closest to us where the medical facility is located, but this location's ADHC is full. It was reassuring to me to see Dad go up to other clients during the visit and talk to them. Also, some of the clients approached us. The doctor told us that Dad would receive a comprehensive health check including an EEG. She may also adjust his medicine after that check-up.

Each morning, I wouldn't leave for school until after Dad had been picked up for his day at the daycare at 8:00. The first day, Julia's back started tensing up before I left and gave her fits all day long. So it was a relief that Dad wasn't home so she could relax some. I called the center mid-afternoon and was told that Dad was well and was having a good time. The driver bringing Dad home at the end of the day had trouble locating the house so Dad was late getting home. I had hurried home to be at home when Dad returned due to Julia's back pain.

When Dad got home after his first day at the ADHC, he was excited and talkative. Julia stated that he looked happier than he had in a while. It is amazing the way God works things!!! We are so grateful that we were able to have some help with Dad. I had dreams of Julia and I taking care of Dad ourselves, but that proved too much, even with assistance from family members. And I don't feel guilty about getting help. Julia had carried the lion's share of the Dad's care while I was in school. It was so difficult for me to concentrate at school knowing how difficult this was getting for Julia. I had taken a couple of half days to be home to help her. At this point, we were slated for Dad to be at the ADHC on Monday, Wednesday, and Friday. If he adjusts well we may go to five days if available. Respite care is also available to us. We are hoping to have some time off during fall break using respite care. It may be too soon to make that happen. Anyway, there is a feeling of relief for us with this all coming together.

Meanwhile, Julia found her birth father's family which has been established by a DNA comparison with Julia's birth father's sister. She is of Creek descent instead of Seminole as Joy and James had been told when Julia was adopted. She was so excited, especially since her adoptive dad, James, had rejected her. She continues to be close to her Joy's family and James's family contacts her often.

As far as the lawsuit, our lawyer attempted to reschedule the depositions with James and Will as the case had stalled. At the first hearing concerning the Temporary Restraining Order and Eviction, we won and James lost. So he couldn't keep us from the house. But with Dad needing our help, we only went to get things we needed from the house. I hope James realized Will had misled him, but James continued siding with Will. There was little cooperation on their part to get the case settled. If they continue to resist, our lawyer is going to implore the judge to order them to comply.

Now that we have help with Dad, we have more emotional reserves to deal with this situation. Without a way to care for Dad, it was difficult to even think about dealing with this. All through this, I have felt that God has intended the lawsuit to take as long as it has for a reason. We keep praying that we have the proper attitude and spirit toward James and Will. We desire that both of them recognize their need for a Savior and they accept God's offer of salvation. That will be worth all of the trouble. So many things happening. God has been so good to us through all of this. We look forward to what God has in store for us each day. Julia and I continue to be close and our relationship to God has never been better. God will make a way where there seems to be no way.

As usual, the school has been busy. There are many new teachers and staff at school with little or no experience. I strive to do my part to support as

Our Struggles With Alzheimer's Disease

many as I can and be an example of what God can do in our lives when we are surrendered to Him. We have so much going on at home, at school, and at church teaching class, and having so many loved ones in church passing, all of it can be draining. Also, with our world growing further away from God, I feel in my spirit that the rapture can happen at any time.

OCTOBER 15, 2021

I am on fall break from school and today is Julia's birthday. I am getting to spend some quiet time with her. Jason's crew (our youngest son) was over yesterday for Chinese food, cake, and ice cream to celebrate Julia's birthday. Only four of them were here due to football practice and work. Anyway, it was a nice quiet time playing Liverpool, a card game, and being together.

We were able to arrange for Dad to be in a memory center for respite care so Julia and I could get some rest. Leaving him there on Wednesday was hard since only family had cared for Dad to this point. Julia had gone with Alisa, a good friend of hers to have a birthday dinner with her. Since Alisa is going to be gone for a few days and will miss Julia's birthday, they are getting together early. So I was going to take Dad to the memory center alone. Julia had made the arrangements since I was working. Earlier in the day, the LifePace doctor gave Dad the complete check which was standard procedure for new clients and I had taken off work to be there. So I had some time with Dad. He returned to the ADHC after the check-up since I returned to work.

That afternoon when Dad got home from the ADHC, I had dinner with him and gave him his medicine. Earlier in the day I had considered calling Jason to see if one of his kids were available to go with me to take Dad to the memory center. Wouldn't you know it, while I was fixing sandwiches for Dad and me for dinner, our youngest granddaughter, Gigi, called and wanted to come to visit! I explained what I was doing and she would go with me to take Dad. It is still amazing to me the way God works!!! It was easier to leave Dad with her there for moral support. We had a fun time driving home on the back roads up to the zoo. Talk about an angel, Gigi was my angel that day!

The ladies who took Dad were gentle and seemed to be patient people. It was hard to drive away watching someone else take Dad to care for him. Due to Covid, I wasn't able to go into the center with him to help him get settled. So I called the next day and Dad was doing fine. I thought of him often during those five days but didn't have any worries or anxiety. I was leery, especially since we tried respite care with Julia's mom when she had Alzheimer's disease and she ended up falling out of a wheelchair the first evening. Then the next morning, the facility sent Julia's mom to the hospital by herself. That attempt at respite care failed. But the way that God has been working things out for us with Dad, I am at peace.

The legal situation with James is starting to move toward a resolution. This day with Dad in respite care is giving Julia and me time to pray, talk, and come to terms with what we need to do. It is a difficult process but still has to be done. Throughout this whole ordeal, God is putting the pieces in place, not always the way we anticipated but He is working in our hearts in ways I never dreamed. We keep praying that God will work in James and Will and Will's wife's lives to bring them to Him. We also pray that we will have the attitude and heart that He wants us to have.

Like last year, I heard it so plainly, God told me that I wanted things to happen that would mess up what He wants to do in my life. His voice in my head was as plain as day. I used to have a lot of worry about this situation, but now I am gaining confidence in trusting God to do something greater than I can do. I pray that our lawyer and others involved will see God shining through us. This whole thing is so heartbreaking to Julia, I feel sorry for her and realize that the best thing I can do for her is to pray for God to give her

His peace. I can be a support for her but I can't change her heart. I don't want her to hold on to any anger or let bitterness build in her. I can't imagine the weight she has to be carrying. She is so strong, stronger than she knows.

Later in the week, the nurse at the memory center where Dad is called to ask about some of Dad's medicine. She assured me that Dad was doing great. He has been waking around 6:00 am. We had reported that he awakes around 6:30 to 7:00 at home. She said he keeps busy and wants to show them what he has done, just like he does at home. I told Julia that I have had peace about Dad being at the center since he has been there. I appreciate all God does for us.

OCTOBER 31, 2021 — A NIGHT IN THE HOSPITAL

Halloween. We were at a friend's house to celebrate our godson's birthday. After we had eaten and were visiting, Dad, Julia, and I were sitting at the table. All of a sudden Dad's head dropped to his chest and I thought that he had fallen asleep, but I couldn't get him to respond. I noted that his lips were blue and his face was ashen and his skin was clammy. He acted like he was going to vomit. He finally came around but was still loopy. This lasted about three minutes. Then he passed out again.

At this point, someone was on the phone with emergency services. Dad stayed in the chair and I held him there. The ambulance arrived fairly quickly. Two young ladies put Dad on the gurney and put him in the ambulance. We gave the information they needed to one of them while the other was working with Dad in the ambulance. None of us were allowed in the ambulance with Dad. The guys drove me to the hospital in our van and Julia rode with Alisa in Alisa's car. At the hospital, only one person was allowed in the waiting room with Dad, so I went with him. Mom, Gary, Charlotte, and Mishelle started toward the hospital. Tina had a house full of people and couldn't come.

Tests were conducted and a decision was made for Dad to spend the night for observation. We were told that Dad was being assigned a room, but he and I ended up spending the night in the emergency room. The rest of the family went home. Many patients had to wait in the hall as there weren't enough rooms available. At least we had a separate space to ourselves. We only received one meal in the 26 hours we were there. Dad didn't sleep any and I only had a hard plastic chair for sitting. And since Dad didn't sleep, I didn't either.

The doctor wanted to conduct more tests the next day and they wanted to further monitor how Dad was doing. The early indicators are that he had become dehydrated. He recently was prescribed lasix and potassium for the swelling in his legs as well as Trazedone. The Trazedone helped him sleep through the night but then he wouldn't awaken when he needed to go to the bathroom. So we did all we could to get enough liquids in him in the early part of the day and not so much after dinner so he hopefully wouldn't have accidents at night. All of this seemed to cause him to be dehydrated.

Still, the doctor checked on his heart, lungs, and brain to be sure nothing was going on there. Anyway, this night spent in the hospital was tough and I hope we never have to do this again. We may have had better luck at one of the hospitals closer to home. Hopefully, we can get these tests done early and get home. Dad is so hard to handle when he is tired like this. He doesn't understand what is happening and why we can't go home.

We are scheduled to have mediation with Julia's dad this week also. Hopefully we can come to an agreement and get this behind us. I truly believe the enemy , satan, is doing all he can to discourage Julia and me. But we will not be defeated!!! We are glad Dad is doing better but I do pray that these hospital trips don't happen often.

Chapter 4

Fall of 2021

NOVEMBER 5, 2021

MEDIATION WENT WELL yesterday. We were able to come to terms with James. We will give him some cash, he will move into Will's house, then we will sell the house. James will need to give us whatever we need to have a clear title to sell the house. A long way from what he and Will wanted. We had no problem giving the money to help James but the driving force behind the lawsuit was Will striving to extort all that he could. He was doing all that he could to make it look like we were taking things from James. But we were striving to keep Will from taking whatever he wanted from James for himself.

We just pray that Will takes care of their dad the way that he should but that is out of our hands at this time. I pray that Julia won't become bitter and that her heart will heal. She has endured a lifetime of torment by Will. The hardest part for her is that James chose to take Will's side over her, basically rejecting her. Dads shouldn't do that. The sad thing is that James would come out far better with us than Will but we can't make that choice for him. Hopefully, Will will now return to their dad what he owes him by taking care of him in his elder years.

We still have my Dad to care for. Not having the emotional strain of this dispute and lawsuit hanging over our heads will be a huge relief. Now to get James moved out so we can get the house ready to sell. Depends on how things go from here as to what we will need to do to sell the house. I know there will be some upkeep that will need to be done.

Through all of this, it has been amazing what God has been doing in our lives! As I have stated before, Julia and I have never been closer. After we finished the mediation, we came home and just cuddled together and decompressed. It was nice to enjoy a little bit of peace from knowing that this may soon be behind us. Later that evening Julia and Alisa went to dinner together as they usually do on Thursday.

My ordination papers came today so I can officiate the wedding of our oldest grandson, Jason, and his fiance'. His dad is our youngest son also named Jason. It is a privilege that they have asked me to perform their wedding. Now I am legal to do that for them. It is so exciting to be a part of this chapter of their lives. I do believe I will be able to marry them in Utah legally also. The plan the kids have is to marry here in Oklahoma with just a small group and then have a public ceremony in Utah. Either way, it will be fun. We just have to make arrangements for Dad. Hopefully, my sisters can work something out so he doesn't need to go back into a memory care center even for a few days. Having Dad stay there is difficult for him and me. I know he doesn't get the care at the memory center that we give him as a family. It is still so good that he enjoys going to the ADHC and that they bathe him there. I still bathe him on Saturday so I can be sure everything is covered. Well, now to concentrate on school work...

November 14, 2021

Yesterday was Dad's 83rd birthday. We had Mexican for dinner then cake and ice cream. Several family members were here and we had a good time.

Tina and Mishelle called since they weren't able to join us, and we talked to Aunt Carolyn. Dad has a bit of a cough and a rough voice. Julia stayed home with him this morning while I taught Sunday School class, and then we watched the church service online together. Dad hasn't slept all morning like he did yesterday. His temperature and oxygen levels are great. Hopefully, his blood pressure will stay strong.

On Tuesday, Dad has a follow-up appointment with the doctor from his overnight stay in the hospital. Some of Dad's medicines were adjusted. I refuse to put Dad through the Lasix routine again. It's too difficult to get him to take in enough liquids and he gets dehydrated. One of the cardiologists who checked Dad was sure that dehydration was the cause of his fainting. None of the tests conducted at the hospital exposed any other causes. One of the medications that was first prescribed to help with pulse control was discontinued. His pulse and blood pressure are staying normal without it. The Namenda was reduced to one dose per day. Trazodone is given at nighttime. I did find that mixing the Zoloft and Trazodone at bedtime caused Dad to be jittery at night time. So one was given at dinner and one at bedtime.

Dad is having more difficulty with things. He requires more help dressing himself. Julia had some Reese's pieces wrapped for Dad's birthday, but Dad wasn't able to get the candy out of the gift bag. Knowing Dad's love of treats, he seldom had trouble getting the wrappers open. Getting to the bathroom, eating, and drinking are becoming more challenging. His right foot gives him pain in the morning, but after he is on it a bit, then he doesn't indicate any problems. His right foot is more swollen than the left. Hopefully, there are no blood clots or anything else going on. All we can do is keep trying.

When Dad doesn't wake up in the night to go to the bathroom, he will wake up wet. I try to get him up at night to take him to the bathroom but often he isn't able to go when I do. Even taking him to the bathroom during the day doesn't always produce results. His bowel movements are erratic. He usually goes every couple of days anymore. When he does it is quite messy. He has gone in his underwear a couple of times, both times with Julia here while I was gone. But such is the way of Alzheimer's disease.

Our lawyer still hasn't received the document needed from James this week. James's lawyer said that he already has the documents they need. Hopefully, that will happen soon. I just pray that Julia's heart will be forgiving. If her dad changes his mind and ways maybe she can be able to have a relationship with him. Now her brother is a different story. We pray that God can get to his heart. He has caused her so much pain. I believe one day that we will be able to have a cordial relationship with her dad. But God is going to have to intervene. That has been the beauty of this whole ordeal, God has done so much for us. I have always felt that God is working on James and Will too.

NOVEMBER 20, 2021

Today we went to a wedding for a couple of young people we know. Dad went with us. The bride was a former student at Rejoice Christian School. It was a beautiful ceremony performed by her grandpa. A real treat for a grandpa. I know the grandpa and had an opportunity to talk to him after the service for a bit. I shared with him that I have never shared this with anyone but Julia that I feel led that I may be called to some kind of ministry after retiring. Not sure what but with today's technology there is now, who knows how that may play out. It may be preaching as lately when I teach my class it feels different at times, like I need to keep sharing instead of pausing for comments or input from members of the class. He offered for me to come to their church on Tuesday nights if I ever want and speak. With Dad at this point, I told him that may not be feasible. This is a bit unsettling to me as I

Fall of 2021

don't know what I need to do. I just wanted to discuss this with an experienced minister. I respect him and his family. I may one day take him up on his offer. I still believe I am supposed to announce my calling to the ministry at Dad's service. I may be getting ahead of God on this. But I believe this needs to be approached with counsel and prayer. I continue to pray.

NOVEMBER 29, 2021

James fell in the shower and broke his hip. He left his phone and emergency button by his bed. He said he crawled for about three hours from the shower to get to his phone and button to call for help. He couldn't get Will to answer his phone. So James called the medics. One of the neighbors saw the ambulance at the house and called me. I was on my way home from work and was still over thirty minutes away, so I called Julia. But Julia had Dad at home and couldn't go. So she called our son, Jason who went out to the house. He got there in time to find out to which hospital James was going. Jason talked to the neighbors who had called me, for a bit and then went to the hospital. With Covid restrictions, Jason was the only one who was allowed in to talk to James.

Jason finally got hold of Will but he was too busy to go to the hospital. From what we understand Will had called James's lawyer attempting to put off moving James as was agreed on during mediation. But it seems that he was told that he still had to move him as stated in the agreement. He didn't want anything to do with James's animals, and from what we can tell he doesn't want James staying in his house. Will told Jason that he would need to build a ramp and a walk-in shower at his house for James. He wants the money we are to give them for the settlement to get this done. James's lawyer told Will that he had to complete the move for James to get the money. We feel sorry for James but he has become untrustworthy for us to want to take on caring for him, especially anything to do with his money. But we don't believe Will should continue to control it, but that is really up to James. There are still a lot of things in motion.

When James fell in the shower he couldn't turn off the water, so it ran for two or three hours and some of the carpet was fairly wet. I went out to the house on the weekend to vacuum up as much water as I was able and to put fans blowing on the carpet to dry out the carpet. I vacuumed three to four gallons of water out of the carpet. I was tempted to pull up the edge of the carpet to aid the drying. I also removed more of our things.

The garage door in the shop needs new springs. I will attempt to do that soon. James has been using antennas for TV but he has plenty of money for cable. So frustrating that it seems that Will has told James that he doesn't have much money. We believe this is so Will can use the money as he wants. We pray that this experience will open James's eyes to Will's lies and deception, from lying about us and to James about how his finances are. Julia and I hope that the truth does come out. Most of all, we also pray that both see their need for God in their lives. God has been SO good to us throughout this whole ordeal.

Out by the pond, a huge branch had broken and was hung up in the Ash tree beside it, finally fell to the ground since I was last out checking on things. That will enable me to be able to clean that area. I had avoided being in that area with the large limb overhead for fear that it would fall on me. Hopefully, over Christmas break, we can get things cleaned up so that we can either sell or move back in. We are now considering selling the house in town and moving to the house Julia's parents gave her. The timing of this couldn't be better as I don't want to pay someone to do this but do it ourselves. Hopefully, the weather will cooperate if this comes to pass. It will be a huge relief to have this behind us. I still believe that God is wanting to accomplish more through this.

Out of the blue, on Friday, Julia got a call from a nurse who was attempting to arrange rehab services for James to enable his broken hip to heal. The nurse told Julia that James had asked her to call Julia. But he said that he wasn't ready to talk to Julia yet. James had told Jason that he was hurt that Julia would steal from him. Again, her stealing from him is not true but something Will has put into his mind. The lawyers, mediators, and others who have seen both sides of the evidence know it isn't true. Hopefully, her dad will see the truth himself.

Julia was so excited that her dad didn't seem to just want to walk away from her. This to me has been one of the most difficult parts of this for Julia. I have always felt that their relationship would be restored, more than likely not to what it had been but the differences would be resolved. I pray that it does. It would be such a blessing to Julia.

Jason is almost to the end of his rope in putting up with Julia's dad's defense of and excuses about her brother. He wants to help his grandpa but Julia's brother is in the way. James, I'm sure, would like to have visits with his grand kids and their kids but he needs to understand that Will doesn't want that and will do all he can to get in the way. If James starts hearing the truth, he may start believing it, instead of the narrative and lies that Will wants James to believe. So sad and frustrating. Jason even told me that eventually, his calls to James's phone go to voicemail.

DECEMBER 13, 2021

Dad has had a cough and obvious chest congestion this weekend. Julia stayed home with him from church. I was hoping that he would be better today, Monday. But he woke up with a fever with his cough and wheezing. I stayed home from school with him today, since Julia already planned to go with Jason to help him. She needs to get out now and then. I am praying that the situation with her dad comes to some sort of ending so we can put that behind us. As hard as it has been, God has been with us through it all and has used all of these circumstances to do some major work in our lives and marriage. It gets very hard sometimes, but God is always good no matter what happens in our lives.

I believe I got the worst of the water out of the carpets at the other house. I am sure we will still need to be treated or change that part of the carpet. There is quite a bit of work and cleaning that house will need before either selling it or moving into it. I believe we would be in a better position by moving into the house and selling this one, but I am leaving that choice up to Julia as she needs to do what she needs to emotionally take care of herself. I hope that I support her as I should. She has been such a blessing to me.

I also feel that God still has something else in mind for us after this chapter of our lives. Not sure what. But it just seems that with the end of time coming and the effort that God is putting into our lives, something seems to be in the works. All I know is God's kingdom is here and I want to be a part in the way that He wants.

CHRISTMAS, 2021

We celebrated Christmas with my siblings and parents at our house with soup and sandwiches. We played Dirty Santa and had a great time. Mishelle and Alan's car broke down and was towed home by Steven, their son, on our trailer. They made it home, thank the Lord. It was good to see Steven and his kiddos. They are growing up so quickly. This was the Sunday before Christmas. Jason's crew was also here except for Jason II, our grandson.

The day before our family Christmas celebration, Julia and I went to meet Julia's biological aunt, her aunt's husband, their son, and another cousin. One cousin lives in Oklahoma, one cousin lives in New Mexico, and Julia's aunt and uncle live in Fayetteville, Arkansas. They are in town picking up Julia's cousin who has flown in from New Mexico for Christmas.

I got pulled over and warned about speeding, doing 71 in a 55 mph zone driving to meet them for dinner as we were running late. Charlotte came to stay with Dad and he started getting sick when she arrived. We still went at Charlotte's encouragement. Not sure what upset his stomach. We often don't know what causes him to suffer various ailments. He was only sick for a little bit. I appreciated Charlotte giving us this time. We were late to dinner as we wanted to be sure Dad was okay.

On Christmas Eve, we grilled steaks, chicken, and brats here since it was in the 70's outside. The only issue was the wind that kept blowing out the flame. We ate and passed out gifts after reading the Christmas story from the Bible in Luke chapter two. Mom and Gary also joined us. They are having difficult times lately also. Then on Christmas day, we stayed home and relaxed. Later that evening we went to our grandson Jason's in-laws for Christmas dinner. They had a smoked turkey and the works! Jason's wife's grandma also joined us. We have known her for several years. We had a great time at every place and event.

During the week since I was off work for Christmas break, we started moving our things out of the other house. James is still in rehab as far as we know. Still no word on moving his things out. I sent our lawyer some ideas to get this done. Since we are going to sell the place, we need to get our things out anyway so it makes sense to take advantage of the time that I have to do so. I know it is a relief for Julia to be doing something.

The carpets seemed to be dry. The animals are doing well as can be. We try to keep the dog out of the house and only in the sun-room, but often the door is left open and she gets in anyway. She chews on so much. Since we keep the upstairs doors closed and now most of our items are out of the house, she only has access to the downstairs when she gets in from the sun-room. We just keep trying. Again, we pray that this week we can get James moved out and finalize the terms outlined in the settlement so we can move on.

The house is a mess. Mice have been through most of the house and the house and garage smell of mice. There are droppings everywhere, even in our stuff. So we are washing everything as we go through things. Our house in town is smaller, so finding room for everything is a challenge. We need to get rid of a bunch of the stuff. The outbuilding has things but these should be easier to clean. I see four categories of things: some we keep, some we burn such as wooden items, the metal will recycle, and then the rest goes to the dump. Whatever is left of value, we will probably send those to be auctioned off. Or we may try to sell it ourselves. We will have to wait and see. Then how to go about selling the house. The market is prime at this time for selling.

I am torn a bit and would almost prefer to move into the larger place for the space. But cutting ties may be easier for Julia. Hopefully, one day we will have a place with more space than we have at the house in town. For now, do we keep the house in town or move to the house where James has been staying?

One other thing, I am considering buying the five years of teaching experience in Alaska into the Oklahoma retirement system. Our IRA money is at an all-time high, so now would be a good time to use some of those funds to buy those years, if the rest of the numbers look to be to our advantage. I almost get the feeling that something will work out financially to allow me to retire early. My concern is that Dad's care is going to increase to the point I will need to be home more but I don't want to leave a financial situation that causes Julia to struggle if anything happens to me. I can easily work another job that isn't so demanding at this point. Teaching school is getting tough with all the other responsibilities I have along with Dad's care. There have been small things that God has been showing me that retirement could happen soon.

I pray that I am a light wherever God places me. I don't want to lose the benefits of the lessons that I have learned during the recent trials of the last few years. God has used all circumstances to better Julia and me for his kingdom and we want to be sure that we ever strive to bring His Kingdom to the world around us. God has helped me overcome some of the most difficult battles that I have waged throughout my life, the heart problems I've allowed to build over the years.

And He isn't finished.... the process will continue until He comes for us, either through death or the rapture. He loves us too much to allow us to go stagnant, but we have to embrace His efforts and not grow hardhearted as Pharaoh did in Genesis of the Bible. What He has for us is so much more than we can envision for ourselves! Read about Job or Joseph also in the Bible. The same God is shaping our lives. He knows what is ahead and will not let us down!!!

Chapter 5

The Beginning of a Pivotal Year

JANUARY 7, 2022

I HAVE BEEN BACK to school for a full week since returning after Christmas break. This is also the first week that Dad was at the ADHC Monday through Friday. Last Friday, Dad developed a rash on his groin. I tried using the Nystatin cream we used for his jock itch in both areas. It seemed to help the rash on his groin but Dad acted like it burned in some areas, so I washed it off of that area. For the rest of the weekend, I kept him washed morning and night. We called the LifePace nurse asking if they would check the area with the rash when he returned on Monday. After the nurse checked him, Dad was prescribed oral medication to help clear up what the nurse described as a yeast infection and also a cream with Nystatin and A&D ointment, one to clear the rash and one to provide a barrier from moisture as Dad now wets himself quite often, especially at night.

I tried getting up each night to take Dad to the bathroom but he usually wouldn't go or be able to go, so I was waking him for no reason. Getting up was also making me tired. Now and then Dad will wake up on his own but not very often. So he is wet most mornings. Depends on how much liquid Dad gets to drink during the day. He gets more liquid when he is home with us it seems. His digestive system is inconsistent. We still give him the Myalax but we never know when he will go. One day last week when he came home from the daycare he had soiled himself but he didn't know it. As soon as he gets home or I get home, I take him to the bathroom right away. If not, more than likely he will need to go during dinner.

He still enjoys his day at the AHDC. I was concerned that going five days would be hard for him, but he is doing well. During the Christmas break, the facility was closed for two days for Christmas and one for New Year's Day. I was home also since school was out for Christmas break for two weeks, so that worked out well. While Dad was at the AHDC, Julia and I spent a couple of days resting and spending time together. Some days we moved most of the rest of our things from the other house. The place was a mess, with mice everywhere as evidenced by droppings. The garage smelled of mice. James's dog and two cats were left at the house. Jason, Julia, and I kept checking on them making sure they had food and water.

I also turned off the water to the house when the temperature was getting so cold to prevent pipes bursting or if they do, prevent flooding. We took water for the animals to drink. One of the patio doors to the sun-room was left open to allow the animals to go outside to use the restroom. I turned the thermostats down so the heat wasn't running a lot, but enough to keep the water in the pipes from freezing. I also replaced the springs on the garage door in the shop as they had broken. I assume the broken springs were the original springs that came with the door.

We are frustrated that we weren't able to finish the agreement with James to get him out of the house. We are sure Will is behind whatever is hindering the process. Jason found out James had been dismissed from the rehab facility but still couldn't get an answer on James's phone. We assume Will may be hoping the animals disappear or get taken so he doesn't have to deal with them. He very likely told his dad that we did something to the animals. No telling with Will. It's just frustrating...

January 14, 2022

Today was different. When I got Dad up for the day, he was all out of sorts. It was difficult to get him to take his medication or drink the water with it the way he usually does. It took about ten minutes instead of the three or so minutes that it takes. He almost couldn't walk by himself and I had to hold him up. He had a difficult time wanting to sit down to go to the bathroom and I almost had to force him to sit. He needed much more help getting dressed. It took over thirty minutes to get ready and into the kitchen. Dad was reaching and grabbing anything like he was nervous or like he was going to fall. Getting him to stand up straight was almost impossible. I had to almost manhandle him to get him anywhere, from chair to chair, off and on the toilet, etc.

He resorts to his sarcastic mood, due to his confusion. It is almost as if he has forgotten how to do many things overnight. I am convinced it is the infection. I decided I was going to stay home from school as Julia will need help with Dad since Dad will be home today due to having a low-grade fever.

We finally contacted someone from LifePace to pick up Dad's urine sample. After we described Dad's symptoms, the LifePace doctor sent an antibiotic even before the results from the sample were completed. We started it right away. Dad also started having a fever. A nurse brought the antibiotic to the house and told us to keep the doctor on-call informed. So I called the doctor with any developments. I also started keeping a log of Dad's vitals. His fever started coming down a bit, which is a good thing. He only ate a banana for lunch. When we had dinner he had a hard time feeding himself. I ended up having to feed him most of what he ate. He had difficulty with one of his medicines which I chopped up and put in his cottage cheese. He said that the cottage cheese tasted differently, but he got it down. I wonder if some of his medications matter at this point. We are afraid that Dad won't regain any of his abilities when we get over this infection. More than likely he won't. I just pray that he doesn't get to the point that he needs to go to the hospital as the last experience was horrible. A specimen was taken by the nurse to be tested for Covid also.

It seems as if the major challenges we face are starting to come together all at once. I have had the feeling that this was going to happen. Hopefully, we will be finished with James finally. That will be a huge load off of our shoulders. My prayer is that Julia will be okay. She continues to stay in touch with her newfound biological family. God has been with us through all of this in so many ways.

JANUARY 15, 2022

Dad woke up with no fever this morning. He seems much calmer and normal. He drank the whole cup of water with his thyroid medicine. He ate his oatmeal by himself and took his other medicine such as his antibiotic. He has trouble standing, but I was able to get him up from the bed and into the bathroom using the walker. It was a struggle getting him off of the stool as there wasn't a lot of room. Dad doesn't like me to lift him or move him and he will fight me trying to get away from me. I don't know how long he would sit if I just left him. I was able to get him to the kitchen with the walker. But the trouble came when I tried to get him to the front room. It took several times and after about thirty minutes we got him into the wheelchair. I wheeled him to the front room and left him in the wheelchair. He has struggled to stand for a while. This will be a challenge...... But God will get us through it.

JANUARY 20, 2022

Well, Dad is walking with a walker and support. But he is unsteady. He is in good spirits and easy to help. Until tonight. As I was trying to get Dad to bed, he started being snotty and I got mad. I left him standing there until he decided that he needed help after all. It took some praying to get things to where he was ready for bed. I know I had to get him to bed and I needed to get away from him to gather myself. I hope Dad doesn't get to be difficult. This is hard enough without him being in a bad mood.

Anyway, he is easier to get around finally. He still has difficulty standing upright at times, just stays bent at the waist. At times he forgets how to move his feet to walk. We still haven't heard if he has passed his Covid test either, so we are still at home one more day. As I was thinking about these things, the thought crossed my mind that the added medicines may be the cause of Dad's problems along with the yeast infection. Too many new variables introduced together... ?? Not sure what it is.

As I sat in quiet time later that night, something I usually do in the morning, God continued to press on my heart. I believe God is using Dad's behavior to teach me another lesson about learning to depend on Him in all things. If God wants to call me to the ministry then He will make the way for me as the need arises. As with all other phases of my life, I didn't have a road map or clear picture of where I would be going or what I would be facing. Throughout my life, God has always brought me through. Some decisions I made or actions that I took could have resulted in crippling or crushing results, if not for God's grace and provision.

My years as a Christian school administrator are a time of my life that has left a significant impression on me in this area. Even our adventures in Alaska are marked with times when it was obvious to us that God was providing for us, at times within hours. There was one twenty-four hour period in which we were able to relocate to Kotzebue after our first year in Alaska. We had four great years in the church in Kotzebue in which God did some amazing things in our lives and where He brought us through some heavy trials.

Anyway, God seems to be impressing me and I need to step out in faith even if doing so seems frightening and unsettling. One of the devotional emails that I chose to read tonight, is one that I had read before and impressed me to the point that I kept it and marked it as unread, so I read it again. It was by a man who had attended our church for a while who pointed out that following God doesn't always make sense or won't always be understood by others, but is rewarding when we obey. He also pointed out many examples in scripture who had done so, Abraham, Moses, and Noah, for example. I don't put myself on their level but their stories are recorded to encourage us to be courageous in following God's directions.

Besides we are coming into a period in our world that Christ's followers are going to need to take a strong stand, otherwise I'm afraid that we will be washed away in the flood of iniquity and false teaching that is eroding the testimony and effectiveness of many Christians. Those of us who have experienced God's goodness need to share our stories so we can encourage others to trust that God makes good of the events of our lives.

I don't know what area or areas of ministry God has in mind for me, but I strongly believe preaching to be an option for the role He wants me to play. Preaching is one of those things that I have said all of my life is something I can't do. I can teach but not preach. Well, never say never.... Then our grandson and his fiance' asked me to perform their wedding, which required me to acquire preaching credentials. Little pieces of the puzzle keep coming together, like one of those puzzles when a piece is added or removed, part of the picture is revealed. So as Julia and I move into the next phase of our lives, we again do our best to step out in faith and trust God to provide as we need. Like He told His disciples, when God tells you not to take provisions with you, God will provide what you need. Even Jesus lived the last three years of His life this way.

Our finances keep pointing to or shaping up to where I can retire and take other employment to make up any difference in what we need. God may not want us to be financially independent but always lean on Him for a part of what we need. I have some dreams that may fill the bill but still require me to depend on God for success, maybe having a gym of my own for older men which can be structured as a ministry as well as helping men to be healthy. Being in business for yourself is one of those things that require God's blessing. We will see...

January 21 & 22, 2022—Friday and Saturday

When trying to get Dad to the table for dinner, we got to the table with the walker and Dad started one of his attitude fits. He was standing with the walker by the counter and wouldn't let go of the walker and started growling and getting angry. I couldn't leave him standing there as he may fall and couldn't get him to let go enough to take hold of the chair to sit down. Julia tried helping me get him to sit down. I tried peeling his hands from the walker which made him even more mad. He resisted and fought against me resulting in him pushing the chair over on its side. The chair being a tall stool, with his momentum and my guidance, he sat down on the side of the chair with a choice word that I had never heard him say before. We left him alone there to cool off where he sat for about five minutes as I continued preparing dinner.

Julia wasn't eating as she had already eaten. I was also angry and needed to cool down, which I did while getting dinner ready for Dad and me. When he started to get up, the chair slid out from under him and he slid to the floor. I was able to get behind him, took his arms, and lifted him off the floor and Julia slid a chair under him. He didn't like it but there was nothing else I could do. He didn't resist this time.

When we sat down to eat, Dad said we needed to get the one who said that out of here. He was referring to the choice word he had said. I told him that he was the one who said it. He was quiet and a bit sheepish. I told him that I had never heard him talk like that. He still tried to blame someone else but I wasn't going to let him get by with that. We finished eating without much talking. He didn't act like he was hurt in any way. After dinner, I gave him the rest of his medicine and took him to the bathroom, but he wouldn't or couldn't go.

That night, I had a little trouble getting his teeth out of his mouth. Eventually, I put him to bed and he was sheepish and apologetic. We read scripture and prayed as usual. Dad slept until 5:00 am when he awoke, but I gave him a melatonin that was lying on his pillow and he went back to sleep. I guess he lost the tablet when I gave it to him at bedtime. I got him up around 7:30. His right arm had a couple of bruises from missing the chair the night before, but he didn't act like anything was hurting.

He had wet the bed thoroughly since he hadn't peed at all during the day before, which was a Friday. He hadn't pooped since Tuesday. He was able to get to the kitchen with the walker after I had dressed him. Thankfully, he was easy to work with and was able to follow directions.

After breakfast, I took him to the bathroom with the walker where he urinated. So I talked with Julia and decided to shower him. The shower went well but was a little more difficult than before, but I was able to give him a thorough cleaning. Then after he ate lunch he finally pooped. It would have been easier to clean him in the shower but I used the wet wipes as I usually do. He was fine the rest of the afternoon.

I left to help Jason for a while in the afternoon. Julia said that while I was gone, Dad started wanting to get up and around now and then. Medicine, infection, whatever it was seems to be causing his difficulties seems to be getting better and Dad is more like himself. However, he does seem to be having some pain in the right side of his chest which he has complained about for a few days. But his vital signs continue to be fine. His blood pressure is lower than normal, but steady. Dad does get winded easily just walking down the hall. As a note, I haven't been giving Dad any coffee for quite a while. He has drank coffee for as long as I can remember but he doesn't seem to miss drinking coffee.

JANUARY 23, 2022 — SUNDAY

Dad is much better. He still struggles to stand and walk. We use a walker and I keep him boxed in with the walker as we walk. I try to get him to walk to the table and the bathroom. It was nice outside so we got in his wheelchair and went up and down the road for a ways. Along the way, he got to see one of his neighbors, who has been a good friend to Dad. Dad has not been able to pee when we get to the bathroom except when it is bedtime. He did poop at bedtime when he tried to pee. I didn't put on his shoes to walk to the bed because there is carpet in the bedroom. He struggled to stand so I could clean him after he pooped. But we worked through it. Now and then he has complained of pain when trying to stand out of a chair. I am praying that he didn't hurt something when he fell on Friday evening.

The best thing is that he is in a good mood and doesn't have the anxiety that he had the last ten days or so. I am more convinced that the antibiotics were the culprit. I doubt that Dad will ever be able to get back to walking on his own, though. With Alzheimer's regaining lost abilities doesn't happen often.

Also, being Sunday we watched several different preachers after watching our church service, which we watched online since Julia stayed home with Dad.

One preacher, David Jeremiah[7] talked about thinking of retirement as an opportunity for continued or increased service in God's Kingdom, something in which I strongly believe. He told the story of one of his parishioners who was a teacher who knew it was God's will for him to retire and begin two ministries in their church, one being a prison ministry that touched many lives. I don't know how many different ways God needs to speak to me. I have talked this through with Julia to let her know what I believe God has for us. I do have one idea to open a gym for older men with a Christian theme and atmosphere. I would like to use the facility to have a place for devotional meetings. I would like to mentor men in their Christian walk as well as their physical health. I believe this could happen after this chapter with Dad is complete. I keep seeking God's will.

I also wonder if there is something that is going to come out of our lives, a book, blog, ministry, etc. to help others deal with hardship, such as caring for aging family members. We aren't sure what, but with the condition of our society today, God is looking for those to step up and minister. I may continue to teach school. Whatever He wants, I want to do my part.

---

[7] David Jeremiah–https://www.davidjeremiah.org/

Chapter 6
We Decide to Move

FEBRUARY 3, 2022

WELL, WE HAVE snow accumulation and again school is on distance learning. It is Wednesday and Dad's ADHC facility is closed Thursday and Friday also. They brought him home today by lunchtime. When the girl who transported him to the ADHC picked him up, I told her we wanted to be sure that he got a shower. The ADHC facility had been giving him showers as he isn't able to get in and out of the tub/shower we have at home since we don't have a walk-in tub. I am so thankful that they can do this for us as well as give Dad a place to go during the day that he enjoys. I told the girl he could come home early today if the weather got bad as I would be here working from home.

The facility called because Dad was resisting taking a shower, but she said the driver told them to call as soon as his shower was over and she would bring him home. I told her that it wasn't my intent for him to come home right away but later in the afternoon. Later they called again to ask if we could pick Dad up around 3:00 as they were short-staffed. I said that I couldn't do that as we don't have a wheelchair vehicle and with ice on the ground I don't want to risk him falling or me getting him in and out of the vehicle. She said that he should be leaving around 4:00. But just before lunchtime, he was home. Julia and I looked forward to having some time alone even if I was working. But he did get showered which was good as it would be quite a few days before he would be going back.

Tonight Dad keeps trying to get up after he went to bed. He hasn't done that in a while. He did stand up on his own from the toilet seat before bed. He stood stooped until I got him to straighten up so I could clean him. I put some ointment on his groin as it was getting sore again. He peed once in the toilet chair but messed in his underwear. At this point, these kinds of things are part of the process and don't frustrate me like they had.

I have learned how to be calm even when he is upset or ugly. It is so hard for him to understand what is happening. He is afraid of falling it seems. He has forgotten how to stand on his own for the most part. He can't walk on his own and can only go short distances with assistance and a walker. With dementia, not many of these abilities will come back. Tonight he keeps sitting on the side of the bed and says he wants to go somewhere but isn't able to get up. I just kept putting him back in bed. I gave him a melatonin hoping that would help him stay asleep.

Usually, I can get him to stand by putting his arms around my neck and hugging him as I lift him. As I get him up, I then have to keep his feet under him and grasp his lower back or backside to straighten him. Once Dad is upright he can usually stand if he has something to hang onto. There have been a couple of times he almost went to the floor. But I was able to get a second grip and pull him on up to the bed or chair. Usually, this is when I need to get his underwear and pants up. I also gave him his calcium pill, which is supposed to strengthen his bones, this morning. We just continue. We have no choice......

I have slipped a little at work, overlooking small things at times, things that I normally have no problem with doing. As Julia and I were talking last night, I told her that it seems that God is pushing me to the point of needing to rely on Him more than on my abilities. My struggle is knowing that I have gifts and things that I can do, but where is that point where God takes over? How does this all fit together? A huge part of the picture is that we do what we can physically, but allow God to change us internally in spirit, emotion, and belief. We learn to do what we do for His reasons and not just to be seen of men. I just want to fulfill His desires for my life.

FEBRUARY 21, 2022

Dad has been getting up and moving quite a bit during the daytime lately. On Saturday when Mom and Gary came to sit with him for a while, Dad got up often and moved around the house. They came to sit with Dad to allow Julia and me to have some time alone. Dad can walk some which is surprising as I stated earlier, Alzheimer patients don't usually regain lost skills. I have him walk from the bedroom to the front room with assistance when we need to move back and forth, just to keep him walking as long as possible.

On one of his forays, he sat on the arm of his chair from the side, then fell backward almost hitting his head on the shelf with his books and things on the other side of his chair. So he was sideways in his chair. Getting him to turn in the chair so we could get him in the chair correctly was difficult. Since moving in this manner wasn't familiar to Dad, he went limp, resulting in him almost sliding to the floor. Julia helped me on one side, but getting hold of him was a problem. Pulling on his arms could cause his shoulder to dislocate and realistically he didn't understand how to help us. I tried to reach down under his hip to get hold of him that way and in doing so my arm pushed in on his side and it felt like his ribs moved to which Dad reacted like he was hurt. My largest fear is that trying to help him, I end up hurting him in the process.

Well, eventually he was in the chair correctly, for the most part, praying about the pain in his side. We let him sit that way for a while. In a bit, I set the chair up fairly high, as the chair is a lift chair, and Dad was able to stand up on his own. I helped him into the wheelchair and rolled him back to his room where we finished the evening activities with no other issues. He didn't give any indication that his side hurt.

At that point, I decided it wasn't a good idea to try getting him into the car for church the next morning, even though earlier that day, Julia and I had discussed trying to take him since he seemed to be doing so well. Getting him in the car seemed too risky. I hate that one of us has to stay home with him instead of going to church together. So I go teach my class on Sunday morning then come home where we watch the service online together. Julia goes to church on Wednesday night, while I stay with Dad. Part of the process.

LifePace is working on getting a lift for us here at the house to help in those instances when Dad isn't able to get himself up. I don't mind lifting him if he isn't agitated or anxious and can work with me. I have had to move him even when he wasn't understanding what was happening. LifePace has been a great group and has been working with us. They are a God send!!

FEBRUARY 27, 2022

We had another week with winter weather, more ice and sleet this time. School was closed Wednesday through Friday and Dad's ADHC was closed Wednesday and Thursday. One of our grandsons, Gabe, was staying with us from Monday to Sunday. It was good to see him. Dad was easy to handle this week. He went to the restroom and got up from his chairs and bed with minimal help. So the week went well. Since he had been going to the day ADHC he was able to get a shower there for which I am thankful. It is getting too risky to get Dad in and out of a car so we haven't gone anywhere with him. We have been trading off church services with one of us staying home with Dad. It doesn't feel the same not going together.

Julia had to pick up Gabe and take him home alone since I needed to be here with Dad and we couldn't get him in the car to ride along. I don't have any hard feelings or feel cheated but it gets difficult at times. Julia also takes it in stride. We do look forward to Spring break when Dad will be in respite care to provide us with some time to rest. I want to take care of Dad myself, but we just aren't able to do it all. We just need to keep him in prayer for the time he is there. With the relaxing of Covid concerns, we may be able to check on him this time. We hope that we can get moved into the other house during the break. It will take some doing and we aren't getting any younger. The Lord will need to give us strength. Julia has decided that she wants to live in the house that her parents gave her and we will sell the other house in town in which we have been living with Dad.

I have found a wheelchair-accessible van for a price we can afford. We will have to borrow the money, but this will make so many things easier. With so many things going on it is difficult to know if this is a good move, but we pray for God's direction. God is so good to us!!

Chapter 7

Spring Break

MARCH 19, 2022

WELL, THE WHEELCHAIR-ACCESSIBLE van didn't work out. The owner it seems sold it to someone else. There must be something else God has in mind. I just pray that tomorrow I can get Dad in the van to get him home after his respite care is over. He has been there for seven days.

This spring break we have been working to get the other house ready. A lot of cleaning needed to be done. Julia wanted to paint most of the walls, especially the paneling in the family room which is so dark. We raised the microwave over the stove top, removed the old wallpaper from the front entry and hall bathroom, and painted the master bedroom and closet as well as the room Dad will use. The place smells a lot better already.

The furnace area in the garage seemed to be the primary nesting area for the mice requiring the removal of wall paneling and replacement of a lot of insulation. There is still a lot of cleaning that needs to be done in the attic and other parts of the house.

Our son, Jason, with two of his boys, Allen, and Logan spent a lot of this spring break helping us with the move. They moved some stuff yesterday, but we didn't have as many things ready to move as we had hoped. We still need to finish cleaning some things at the house and then organize our stuff to be moved. The difficulty is that I go back to school on Monday and will not have much time to help. Several people have helped us. Alyson and her friend helped with the cleaning also.

Jason, our grandson Jason, his fiance, Maci, and our granddaughter, Gigi helped some on Friday. One of the men from our church and his daughter helped for two days. A lady from our Sunday School class helped Julia with cleaning for a couple of days. Another friend of Julia's helped with cleaning. We have been so thankful for all the help.

I have wanted to go check on Dad while he is in respite care since I am allowed, but we have so much that we need to get done to prepare to move that I want to use the time for that purpose. Besides, on Sunday we went down to Hatfield, Arkansas, for Aunt Carolyn's funeral which was Monday morning. Aunt Carolyn was Dad's sister. So we weren't able to use those two days to work on the house. It was good to spend time with Tina and Mishelle as well as Aunt Carolyn's family. It was while attending Aunt Carolyn's funeral that Charlotte and I had a conversation about Dad's funeral.

Then this week my uncle, the husband of one of Dad's other sisters, passed away. His service is this Monday, March 21st. I don't see how we can make it to this service. Dad will be back with us and I will be starting back to school. Dad is the most difficult hurdle to get around. I will just have to send my condolences as much as I hate doing it that way.

MARCH 20, 2022

Well, Julia and Charlotte are going to our uncle's funeral to represent our family tomorrow. I will take care of Dad. Hopefully, Dad's ride to the ADHC won't be too late. Julia and Charlotte will leave here around 7:30 am. Then I will need to hurry home from school to be here when Dad gets home.

Spring Break

Today, Sunday, I picked him up from respite care at 2:30. When I went into his room at the memory center he was ready to go. He teared up a little when I told him we were going home. One of his shoes was missing and took a while for the staff to find. There are a couple of clothing items missing, but we left without those.

On the way home, I stopped to get hamburgers for dinner for us. Now and then I get Coke for Dad to drink as he likes it. He only drinks a little bit anymore, so I don't get Coke for him often. I also gave him some coffee after dinner, another of the things I don't give him often. He is bad about letting it sit and get cold. Getting him to drink any liquids at all is difficult. When we were headed home, he said that he was thirsty so I gave him some water that we had in the van. He was talkative as I expected that he would be. He has some bruises on his arms but it doesn't take much of a bump or scrape to cause a bruise.

One day during the week he was in respite care, and a nurse called to tell me that Dad had gotten out of his chair, falling and getting a cut on his arm. There was still a bandage on his arm so I wasn't able to see the injury as it was stuck quite well. It may come off when he is in the shower tomorrow. But I may try to soak it off when he gets home. Today I spent time trimming his ears, beard, eyebrows, cheeks, etc things we usually do on Saturday.

He was easy enough to get into the van to come home from the nursing home. One of the staff members came out and helped me get him out of the chair. It was easy enough to get him in the van as he didn't fight me and let me more or less lift and move him to where he needed to be. And getting out of the van was easy. After we were in the house, I had to lift him out of the wheelchair to move him into the easy chair, and then again to to get him on the bathroom chair. Then he stood up on his own from the bathroom chair and used the walker and my help to walk to the bed. We went through

What I Learned From Dad

our normal routine as he was tired and almost fell asleep in his chair. I was glad that he was home.

He said his room looked nice, but I don't know if he remembered that it was his room from before. I showed him pictures of family members we often talk about and moved the picture of his mom and dad and one with his siblings by his bed for him. I think he was happy to be home. I told him I was sorry I had to have someone else care for him so I could have a break and get the other house ready. I believe Dad is no worse for wear. I prayed for him throughout the week. I considered going to visit him during the week but was afraid that he would be disappointed that he didn't get to leave with me. Besides we had a lot to do, and I knew this was short term, so I didn't go. It may have been the wrong choice, but that is what I did. All of this is so tough. I just pray that we do the right thing.

Still, no luck finding a wheelchair-accessible van. I will need to keep looking. If this is what God wants us to have, He will help us find it. This has been quite a learning experience.

MARCH 23, 2022

Julia had a routine mammogram last week, then was informed at the end of the week that she had a cyst on the left side that they wanted to ultra scan. She went in today and it was as if the cyst had disappeared. We thank God for His sustaining care of her. To Him be all the glory! So all is well.

Dad is getting his spunk back after being in respite care for spring break. I hated to have him there but we needed to have some time to work on the other house and to have a chance to take a break for rest. He also has some bruises from falling. We were called about one of the falls when he gashed his arm. Even LifePace noticed the bruises and seemed to think there were quite a few. Hopefully, we won't need to use respite care very often. Charlotte is coming to sit with Dad on Sunday when we have a special

Spring Break

service at church, a young family who we support in their missionary work. There is a lunch with them at church after the service we want to attend. We appreciate that Charlotte is willing to do this for us.

MARCH 31, 2022

Tomorrow is April. Wow, where has time gone? Dad has seemed to have rebounded from his stay in respite care. I appreciated the time to get a lot of things done. He has had a problem with constipation but things seem to be working out. The skin under his beard is red and irritated beyond what I realized, but I am working on it. If necessary, I will trim his beard shorter or shave it. He has had his beard so long that he would look strange without it.

We also just found out that Dad's ADHC will be closed on Monday. We didn't know until the driver told us that she saw a sign at the front desk as she was dropping Dad off. So I will need to take the day off. Mom and Gary probably won't make it over this weekend to sit with Dad so Julia and I can get a break. Gary is having trouble with his knee. It seems that it is going to take forever to get into the other house.

This Friday is Good Friday and Dad's doctor appointment is that morning. Julia went to that appointment with Dad that day so I could keep getting things ready so we could move.

But this Monday I need to stay home with Dad since the Adult Health Care facility is closed. It happens to be a Professional Day at school so I won't have to have anyone cover my duties. That helps. I do enjoy those days at school as we can get a lot more done without the students at school. It will be nice if we can move and then sell this house in town and have money to do some things that we want to do and only be responsible for one place instead of two places.

Also, there is a gospel singing this week but we won't be able to attend. If we had a van with wheelchair access so we could take Dad we could go. He

April 14, 2022

Well, we plan to make the move to the new house this weekend. It is Easter weekend and Gary's birthday. I have tomorrow, Good Friday, off of work and Dad can go to his daycare so we can have time to get some things done to prepare for moving. We have some help coming on Saturday. There is a chance of rain, but hopefully that won't happen. We won't be able to get everything moved but enough to start living in the other house and prepare the house in town for selling. We want to have a garage sale at the house in town to get rid of a lot of stuff. Since the house is in town, there is more visibility for having a garage sale.

Since Dad's dentures are becoming loose, a dentist attempted to either alter Dad's dentures or make him a new pair but wasn't successful. Dad has no lower gum line left for his dentures to grip. We will have to do the best we can with what Dad has. We will just need to be sure he has soft food. It was hard to watch Dad struggle to understand the directions of the dentist as he attempted to get an imprint of Dad's gums. Some of the material used to make an imprint of Dad's gums got stuck in his beard and mustache and I did my best to remove it with minimal pain. The material became a hard rubbery substance that stuck in his whiskers so that I either had to pull the material out of his beard or cut his whiskers. Either way, it was painful for Dad.

Dad was so tired. He almost fell asleep during one part when he had to sit still in an attempt to get an imprint. When he arrived at the dentist from the ADHC, he was chewing something that looked to be chicken. I had him spit it out and threw it away. This is the reason we were at the dentist as he isn't able to chew very many things. All to no avail, we will just have to do the best we can with the dentures he has.

Spring Break

Tomorrow Dad has his annual physical. So I will leave school and go to the doctor's office for that. I also got a new CPAP machine due to a recall on the one I currently have.

The last few weeks have been a whirlwind getting things ready to move. The house was a mess. Even after we get in, we will have to fix things. But it is clean enough for Julia to feel it is ready for us. She has been a trooper and working so hard! She has lost some weight and been so tired at times. Still struggling with getting enough sleep every night. She doesn't complain of hip pain and back pain as much. I believe having to sit so much as we were caring for Dad caused a lot of her pain. I may be wrong but she hasn't complained very much. She is building stamina which had diminished. She does seem more at ease and like she has a purpose. We still don't know for sure what to do with a lot of her dad's stuff that was just left behind. Hopefully, we can get that settled soon and get James's stuff out one way or another. It smells so much like mice. Those little creatures had taken over the place. Julia has done a great job of clearing those out.

Gary and Mom haven't been over much, Gary is having problems with his knee. It is one thing after another with that boy. I don't guess Mom will drive the pickup as it is a standard. Her car isn't drivable.

We wonder how the move will affect Dad. He seems so tired most of the time. He sleeps about twelve hours a night. He enjoys the time at the ADHC but it wears him out. He is ready for bed almost as soon as he gets home. So we eat together then I get him to bed. The other night he got up a couple of times during the night, so I got him on the pot and he peed. Then he went back to sleep and stayed asleep.

Also this week one morning as I had him up to pull up his underwear and pants, I asked if he needed to go to the bathroom. He said, "Yes" so I went for his portable toilet chair. Before I could get him set down he started going while standing, both of them. He has peed a couple of times as I was getting him ready, but never both. Thankfully, I had a disposable pad on floor under him just in case. Nevertheless, it made quite a mess even if the pad caught the mess. I cleaned him and changed him. From now on, I will have the chair by the bed ready when he wakes up, just in case. Just part of the process.

APRIL 24, 2022

The last week and weekend have been busy. I had Good Friday off of work so we moved most of the large items to the big house. We weren't intending to do that on Friday but on Saturday. We planned to box up as much as we were able on Friday to be ready to move it all on Saturday. Our bed was the major large item that had to be moved on Saturday. We are using the twin bed Charlotte gave us for Dad. We will probably sell his bed or possibly move it upstairs in the new house just in case.

Dad seems to have settled in and has no problem using the smaller bed. He asked me one time yesterday when we were going home. This place doesn't feel the same to him, actually it doesn't feel the same for any of us. Julia has been working so hard and I am proud of her and all that she has done. Only twenty more days of school and I will be able to help more.

We have a lot of stuff in the house to go through. We are not too sure what to do with all that was left here of James's stuff. It takes up a lot of room and most of it smells like mice. So most of his stuff is in the shop. We have cleaned what we want to use. Even to sell the stuff in a garage sale we will have to clean it. It will be nice if we can get through the final paperwork with James and have this behind us. We assume that he doesn't want any of what was left. On the day that was scheduled for James to get his things from the house, only Will, his wife, and the movers came to get James's stuff. I assume James listed what he wanted and that is what was taken. Then the rest was left for us to handle.

The foodstuff left in the house seems to have those bugs that turn into moths that lay more eggs. Gross things. A lot of it is hard on Julia with all of the emotions that are involved in what was done to her. She gets overwhelmed at times because there is so much to do. Even if she sits to rest it stresses her seeing things piled up. I try to hide what I can so she can deal with it when things settle down and we aren't so stressed. Also, I try to do all I can to complete the tasks that I can to help. With schoolwork, though my time is limited. We are taking time this Sunday afternoon to rest.

On Thursday night, the 21st, our grandson, Jason, was married to Maci. It was a nice wedding. It was at a place in Broken Arrow. They wanted to hold the ceremony outside with a small group of guests. They had dinner for us, chicken fried chicken with mashed potatoes and green beans, and cheesecake for dessert. I was so excited and honored that they had asked me to officiate their ceremony. I secured my ordination papers from a foundational church in Dallas, Texas that provides the service for situations like this. This church only promotes traditional marriage between one man and one woman. There are many "churches" that provide ordination services for same-sex marriage, so I avoided those organizations.

To enable Julia and I to go to the wedding, Charlotte came and sat with Dad. She had just gotten out to the lake for her first night of camping. But she had committed to watching Dad before she planned her trip, so she came anyway after getting her camp ready. We appreciate her doing this for us.

The ceremony was nice. A little windy, messing with the veil and the pages of my Bible and notes. But we got through it. I had been praying that I wouldn't become emotional or make any major goof-ups during the service. I basically read my script but did my best to look up now and then to make eye contact with the young couple and the audience. I focused on projecting my voice to be heard, emphasizing important points, and everyone said they could hear me well when I asked some of those attending after the ceremony. So I felt good about how things went. One of my granddaughters said that she wants me to do her service when the time comes. But I told her that would be awhile as she still is so young, but being asked is an honor. Everyone said they had a good day. The wedding was a small intimate group. A reception is scheduled for later in June is a big celebration that will have a large group.

I have arranged to have a Horstman family reunion in June. Our family has had this event for several years around this time of year. Dad and his youngest sister are the only siblings in their family that are left. Since Dad isn't able to travel, we decided to host the event here. Not sure how many will come. I have reserved the church gym and cafe for the reunion. I hope that I can get Dad there and back. If needed we can have everyone at our house. We do have room if we are outside. We should have the house in good order by then. But the church has a gym for the kids to play, tables and chairs for eating, and is indoors in case it rains or is too hot to be outside which will be much better. I also created a private Facebook group to share pictures and invite people to the get-together. I hope we have a good turnout.

Mom's 80th birthday is this week. We will celebrate on Saturday at our house. We are having Italian food which is Mom's choice. One of our daughters-in-law, Hayley, is making a chocolate cake with chocolate icing a favorite type of cake of my family. We ate many such cakes as kids. I hope Mom has a good birthday. Gary found a cabinet for Mom to display her collection of small bells. Together we, her kids, bought as a birthday gift. We are individually getting bells for her to add to her bell collection. Gary's knee has been hurting him. Hopefully, he can get Mom here next weekend and also attend.

Last of all, we have had different people ask about buying our house in town. I just hope that the foundation isn't a problem with all of the piers we had to install. We are being upfront with everyone about the piers. One neighbor's brother wants to buy the place for as little as possible, but of course, we want to get as much as we can. Another family is from Washington state and has put in offers on fifteen places in the area but has lost all of them to other bidders. Our house has a lot to offer, but we are not sure how to proceed. We would love to avoid the fees of a Realtor but we don't want to make any major mistakes. Selling that place would enable us to do what we would like to renovate the other house. We still have so much to move and no place to store stuff. My shop things will probably have to be put in the shed until we can get the shop organized. There is a mess in the shop. But we will get there..... Just a lot is happening right now.

APRIL 27, 2022

Dad has difficulty eating things unless the food is soft or ground up. He loves peanut butter and jelly (PBJ) sandwiches so we give those to him often. He likes apple sauce and bananas. The center at LifePace called and said he wasn't eating a lot there and he has lost weight. He was 169 pounds six months ago and at his last doctor appointment, he was 151 pounds. So they are going to give him Ensure, a protein drink with added vitamins, with his meals at the center to see if he will drink those.

He eats well with us, usually eating oatmeal for breakfast and a banana. Then he usually eats what Julia and I have for dinner. If the food is hard to chew Julia will chop it up or substitute it for something he can eat. Cottage cheese, macaroni and cheese, rice, green beans from a can, peas, eggs, burger, etc.. He is still able to feed himself for the most part. It is getting to the point where I have to put his pills in his mouth to get him to take them. Getting him to drink enough water is still a struggle. I give him a little coffee now and then to get as much liquid in him as possible. I'm not sure if the caffeine will affect his sleep at this point, but caffeine hadn't affected his sleep before he started exhibiting symptoms of Alzheimer's disease.

I have to lift him more often to get him to stand. The positive is that he doesn't fight me as much and doesn't seem as afraid. And he isn't as heavy as he was which sadly makes it easier.

Dad woke up at 4:00 am this morning. I think he was chilly so I put another blanket on his bed. I got him back in bed, gave him a melatonin and he slept until I got him up. I don't believe he went to sleep right away. Boy was he tired. He went to bed ready to sleep tonight. And he went to the bathroom before he went to bed. It is much easier to clean him at that point than it is if he soils himself in his sleep. And I feel better when he doesn't sleep in the stuff. It's bad enough that he sleeps in urine most nights. This disease is ruthless! I hate it and what it does to him.

Last of all, Mom's birthday is Friday and we celebrate here on Saturday. That is due to Dad not being able to get in and out of a car preventing us from going to Mom and Gary's place. It would be easier for Mom and Gary to have her birthday at their house. Anyway, I hope it goes well.

MAY 10, 2022

Dad was taken by ambulance from the ADHC as his blood pressure went high and his pulse rate went low. By the time he was in the emergency room, he wasn't having any problems. The hospital ran the basic tests and all came back normal, so they sent him home.

Julia called me right after the ADHC called her to inform us that Dad was en route to the hospital, so I left school to meet the ambulance with Dad at the hospital. After the ER staff determined that there was no reason for Dad to stay at the hospital, one of LifePace's transport vans came to get Dad and take him home. So we both just went home for the rest of the day.

Chapter 8

Life in the New House

MAY 15, 2022

WE ARE SETTLED in the house and are preparing to sell the house in town. Julia has been working hard to get things organized to have a garage sale before we sell the house. We are also working to get this house in shape. I used about two gallons of insecticide in the house because we have seen spiders throughout the house and other bugs in the food. We despise those things! I am sure I will need to spray again in about ten days. It will be easier to do with Dad at the ADHC and me out of school since school is out on May 20th. I have a lot to do to be ready to check out for the school year, but I should be able to get everything done by the last day. We have so much to do right away. And there is the Horstman family reunion on June 11th at the church. We are always so busy.

Dad was a bit of a challenge part of the day. He couldn't remember how to stand up to go to the bathroom at noon today and got snarky when I lifted him out of the chair to put him on the toilet. It took him a bit to get on his feet. Even Julia stepped in to encourage Dad and he snapped at her. He was growling and giving me smart-aleck answers. He did pee but that was all. He and Julia sat outside while I sprayed the house. We waited for an hour for the insecticide to dry before going back into the house. I used the one-and-a-half gallons that we had, so I had to get more. I still can't believe the condition of the house and what Julia's dad lived in.

Last weekend, I spent about three hours vacuuming a lot of the insulation out of the attic around the furnace and garage area where the mice had done their nesting. The insulation in the attic was so contaminated with mice droppings and urine that the smell would drift down to the garage, especially on a hot day. I was concerned that the odor would become overwhelming when the summer heat began. So I vacuumed three large trash bags of insulation from the areas where there were signs of mice nests. One of Julia's mouse blocks of repellent had some bites so at least one or two are around. The shop where the stuff from the house is stored smells of mice, even worse on hot days. We look forward to having all of this clean. The first order of business is to get the other house ready to sell, then work on getting this place as we want it.

It's still a mystery why we haven't heard from James about settling everything, especially since it is obvious the case is a lost cause. The settlement cash is there for them. Oh well, such is life. I would love to never give the cash to them, especially since we assume James will probably pass it on to Will.

One of our granddaughters graduates from high school on Tuesday. Mom and Gary are coming over for that. Mom is going to the graduation with us and Gary is going to sit with Dad. I am taking the last half day of personal leave I have left to come home early to help Julia a bit at the other house before we go to the graduation. Then Dad is to come home early from the ADHC so I can get him ready for bed a little early for Gary. This will enable us to get to the graduation as early as possible. We appreciate Mom and Gary doing this. Mom hasn't been to many of the kid's things lately with them being so far away. Gary's knee is acting up and giving him a lot of pain. I know his knee hurts a lot as well as his back. We are grateful for their help.

Julia is helping one of the neighbors with his garden and planting some things for us there. We still have asparagus coming up from the bed we started a few years ago. I was surprised to see the asparagus since we haven't been here to cultivate it. The neighbor Julia is helping had maintained the garden with his wife, but she passed away almost two years ago. So it is good for him to have Julia there with him. Julia is learning a lot from him about gardening also.

I plan to put a new bridge over the creek that connects our backyard to our field since the first one washed away. I have a couple of long pieces of pipe for building it. Julia is ready for it to be there now. She saw a snake the other day and she would like a clear place to cross the creek. So I took the weed eater and cleared a large section of the creek bank for her until I could get the bridge built. It will be nice to have a clear place to cross without going down into the creek.

Things are slowly coming together, it will be nice when have things like we want them. Things will go quicker when I get out of school. I'm not as young as I used to be and not being able to be as active the last four years with caring for Dad has slowed me down a little. My arms and hands give me the most pain. I'm sure it is a carpal tunnel issue. But I don't want to slow down enough or take the time to treat it. And I wouldn't be able to deal with Dad if I ended up having surgery. I am just thankful God has blessed me with the health and strength that I have. God has been so good to me in so many ways. I can't be thankful enough!

I got a speeding ticket about ten days ago. I guess I was about due. I was driving the same speed as almost everyone else on the highway and for some reason I was stopped. I guess it was my turn. Oh, well.... I'll pay the fine and move on.

Chapter 9

Beginning of the End

May 16, 2022—Sunday morning

WHILE I WAS teaching my Sunday School class at church today, Dad was home with Julia. Dad tried to get out of his wheelchair on his own and he fell breaking his right femur up by his hip. Julia couldn't get me to answer my phone as I had my phone on silence since I was at church. And I didn't sense the vibration of the phone, which was activated. She called 911.

It just happened that LifePace had arranged for a ramp to be installed at the house to wheel Dad's wheelchair from the ground level to floor level. The man installing the wheelchair ramp was at our house on Sunday as he had a family emergency and hadn't been able to install the ramp until today. Julia stepped out a minute to talk to him and in that little bit, Dad fell. I felt bad that I didn't see her text or hear her phone call until after I finished teaching class and was getting in the car to come home. She was able to ride in the ambulance with him. I called her right away and we were able to talk on the phone while she was riding in the ambulance. I got behind the ambulance after leaving church and I followed them to the hospital.

It took a while for all things to come together at the hospital due to a staff shortage and the Covid issues, but soon it was determined that he definitely broke his hip. Conditions at the hospital weren't as bad as the last time Dad and I spent the night at the hospital. He will probably have surgery the next day. After the surgery he will be in the hospital for a day or two then he will be taken to a rehabilitation (rehab) facility until his hip is stable enough for him to be cared for at home. I'm not sure how things will go with the rehab and his having Alzheimer's disease. I hate that this happened when I wasn't at home. I don't want Julia to feel bad, but you never know when Dad will try to get up as he has been so unpredictable.

I still have one week of school to go. Julia may be able to sit with him at the hospital some of the days so I can finish up what I need at school. I hate being gone from school during the last week as things get so busy. I have most of my paperwork done though.

I keep having the feeling that this will be the last summer we will have with Dad. He is getting so frail. I don't want him to get to the point that I can't take care of him and his last days are with strangers. I don't believe that is the way it should be. Hopefully, LifePace can provide what we need so that he can stay at home, if it comes to that point. I'm afraid that this incident will bring him closer to the end of his life.

God has confirmed in so many ways that this journey has many aspects that benefit me. God has taught me so many things and blessed Julia and me during this time of taking care of Dad and navigating other challenges, such as:

- the whole mess with James and Will coming to an end,
- me working full-time,
- seeing Julia work through the emotional issues of all that happened to her,
- then finding Julia's biological family and find out her biological dad lived close by all these years,

- Mom, me, and my siblings have grown closer,
- Julia and I are growing closer to each other and closer to God as a couple,
- each of us individually growing closer to God.

I'm not sure what to do about the Horstman family reunion coming up soon. It looks as if Dad will not be able to attend. Dad's sister already said that she probably won't make it. I think attending at this time will be too hard on her being the only sibling, especially if Dad isn't there. She told me that she took a fall herself and landed on her face and is recovering from that. Poor thing! But I will probably go ahead and host the event for the ones who want to get together. There are quite a few of us cousins who have been fairly close to each other throughout the years. This will be one last time we can be together as the Horstman family with Dad. We will see how it goes.

MAY 17, 2022

Dad has surgery to fix his hip at 3:30 today. All Dad wants to do is get out of here, which I would love to do with him. He is done with all the poking, prodding, and being bothered by the hospital staff. I would feel the same way. I feel like a parent caring for a child. It is traumatic for him also. He doesn't understand. He doesn't trust me as much as he did since I help the doctors and nurses do things that hurt him. He doesn't understand that these things are necessary to treat his break and hopefully help him get better. His whole world seems to be against him. Poor guy, I feel so sorry for him.

He will be in a rehab facility for a while after the surgery. I had been considering making arrangements for more respite care, but that doesn't look necessary now. I have spent time reviewing facilities online to decide on a skilled care rehab facility for Dad after the surgery. All of the facilities that are approved by his insurance are in south Tulsa, about 30 minutes from our house. I want to see him three or four days a week at least. At least the Covid restrictions have been lifted. I hope the fact that he hasn't taken the Covid vaccine doesn't make a difference to them. Crazy world. His insurance will pay for skilled nursing instead of rehab which will be better. I finally made my choice.

MAY 18, 2022

Dad is a lot better today. The surgery has helped. The Physical Therapist was able to get Dad to sit up without him acting like it was painful. He wouldn't stand. She tried different ways to get him to stand. I told her that is what I go through everyday, even before he fell. She was going to set him in the chair but gave up. She finally settled him back in bed. He didn't act like anything she did hurt him. I was surprised. He did react like it hurt when she and the tech put the pillow back under him after he was back in bed. She didn't want me to help, but for some reason she went to get one of the staff. I did get up to hold his hands when he kept grabbing at her as she tried to push the pillow under him. Then I lifted his leg to put the pillow under it. The pillow was to keep him from laying on the same part of his backside. He slept for a while after that. He was given some Tylenol and he drank almost two Boost protein drinks and ate a small amount of his breakfast. He slept more after that.

Around lunchtime, he ate a little more and drank a small amount of an orange Boost with Miralax added. He ate a little of his lunch. The dietitian came around and told me to give him all the protein he would take as this would help with the healing process. The surgeon also came by to see how Dad was doing. He seemed pleased. He said he is fine with Dad going to a skilled nursing facility this week. The hospital doctor came by again as she has each day.

The case worker said my first choice of a skilled nursing facility didn't have an opening this week. She asked which facility was my second choice. I told her the other facility I preferred. Hopefully, something will open soon. Dad has done much better than I anticipated.

Charlotte is staying with Dad tonight at the hospital so I can rest and go to school for a while tomorrow. I feel better now that Dad is past the worst. And I need to get some things done at school. Julia will stay with him for a while after Charlotte leaves so I can stay at school a little longer if needed. I appreciate both of them doing this. I need a shower badly and I am tired. Dad was ready to get up and go with me. I felt sorry for him because he didn't understand anything happening to him.

MAY 19, 2022

Dad is settled into the skilled nursing facility. We were able to go in and help get him settled. He still had some of the hospital blankets with him, which I returned to the hospital later. The arrangements and his being moved happened more quickly than we anticipated. I was in school at the time, so I left school to go with him when Julia called to tell me he was being moved. Julia and Charlotte were already there at the hospital with him. The three of us met the ambulance at the facility. Hopefully, things will go well and Dad can get better.

MAY 20, 2022

My last day of school for the year!! I went by to see Dad after school was out. He seemed to be doing well. The nurse said he sat in his wheelchair for several hours today by the nurse's station. Then he took an afternoon nap. But he isn't eating a lot. I tried to get him to eat and he ate some for me. Not as much as if he were at home, but more than a couple of bites that the nurse said he had eaten for them.

I got him to eat on his own for most of the time but fed him some of the applesauce. The doctor saw him today and ordered some standard blood tests for patients coming into the facility. She said the doctor told her that he fought when the blood was drawn. I spent over an hour with him trying to get him to eat more. Then I turned the TV onto Mash which we watch most evenings before he goes to bed. I read some scripture with him and prayed with him. He seemed to be fine.

When I was getting ready to leave, Dad wanted to come with me. I tried to tell him off and on that, he had to stay until his hip was well enough for him to be at home. I don't know how much he understands. It was hard to leave him again. Knowing we would be there tomorrow helps. I hope some of the siblings can make it. They also said that we could bring one of Dad's long-handled spoons that he used at home to help him eat. He has a hard time eating with the short-handled spoons they had.

I tried one more time to get his teeth in. Like yesterday, he put them in part way then took them out. He seems to think he will choke on them. He may never get them back in. I also used the small scissors on the Swiss army knife I had in my pocket to clip the hair to remove one of the electrode patches left on his chest from the hospital. He fought me and I only got one off as it was difficult not to pull his hair some while cutting the hairs, so I didn't attempt to remove the other electrode patch. I didn't want to cause him any more discomfort than needed. I almost sense that Dad is giving up. This is all so hard.

MAY 29, 2022

Julia, our granddaughter, Gigi, and I went to see Dad today after taking a washer and dryer set to Mom and Gary. We have also heard the news that Mom's brother who lives in Wyoming is going to pass away at anytime. My Uncle's cancer has come back with a vengeance. He has had one chemo treatment but that didn't seem to go so well so he decided against having any other treatment and to let nature run its course. Of course, Mom was broken-hearted but she was able to talk to him today on a video call, and that made her feel better. He also told Mom that he would see her in a better place, which made her feel that he had given his life to God since he would never tell her that before. This is assuring for all of us. Charlotte went over last night to spend the night with Mom. She said Mom is much better today. So that is good. Charlotte and her husband are working on flight arrangements for Charlotte and Mom to go to Wyoming. I would like to go, but I need to be here for Dad.

Dad was really in a lost state the last two days. He talks a lot but none of it makes sense. He reaches into the air for things that aren't there. At times he acts like he is putting something in his mouth. One thing that was different this time, at one point he reached for me and hugged me. This is something that he rarely did as he didn't show emotions often. He still talks about being ready for Heaven, talks about Jesus often, and at times talks like he is talking to Jesus. He will stop and pray with us but doesn't respond to many other things. At times he acts like something hurts. It's hard to know if he is hurting or just uncomfortable. I rubbed his back for a while which seemed to help.

We were finally able to have a garage sale at the house in town this weekend. We had a lot of rain and the ground was soft, so Jason, one of our grandsons, Allen, and I got the truck stuck at the other house getting plywood sheets to use for table tops to set out garage sale items. We carried the plywood sheets to the van to transport them to the house in town. That was on Thursday. I was able to drive the truck out Saturday after the ground dried a bit. On Friday, I winched the truck out of the ruts with a hand winch so I had no problems driving the truck out of the muddy spot.

Saturday was the busiest day for the garage sale. But it rained a couple of times and when we pulled everything in the garage around noon. The second time it rained after we had set things back out, we ended for the day.

Preparing for a garage sale is a lot of work and we were tired. We decided to try one more time next weekend. We will work during the week to get the rest of the things out of the shed and house moved so all we have left to do is to get rid of what remains from the garage sale after we sell all that we can. Then we can sell the house. We don't know whether to sell the house ourselves or use a Realtor. The Realtor will get a large chunk. But we want the sale to go smoothly. Most of all we want to follow God's will. Selling it on our own, we will need to hire an attorney to make sure we do all things correctly. So, either way, we will need some guidance and there will be an expense.

Also, our attorney told us that the paperwork to finish the mediation agreement with James is almost complete. A lot is currently happening. It will be nice to have this cloud from over our heads. Getting the settlement money together will be a bit of a challenge. Then we want to help pay for Mom's plane ticket to Wyoming. Selling the house will solve a lot of our current problems. But God is in control and He has given me peace about all things. We do our best to keep in touch with God so we make the correct decisions.

This whole thing is wearing us down physically and emotionally. I have even taken a couple of naps which I don't do regularly. We can't wait until we get through this chapter of our lives: spending time with Dad while taking care of moving, getting settled into the house, settling the lawsuit with James, etc. At least I don't have to worry about school since it is summer break, that helps a lot.

We decided not to have the family reunion with the Horstman family. There is too much to do to put things together and I am emotionally drained with Dad being as he is. I had planned this reunion because it may be the last one that Dad may have been able to be a part of. Now that he isn't able to attend my heart isn't in it. There is always next year.

June 1, 2022

Where did last month go?! Here we are in June. The weather hasn't been hot yet. We have had some warm days but more cooler days than it seems we usually have at this time of year. We've had quite a bit of rain and are supposed to get more tonight. That was the case today, but not much fell. I hurried to do what I could before the rain came but the rain didn't arrive. Julia and I emptied most of the large things from the shed at the other house. I hope to have everything out of the house by the end of this week. We have had different people look at the house interested in buying it.

After visiting with Dad this morning, I spent most of the evening trying to clean the chairs from the house that will possibly sell. They still smell a bit but look better as we had been trying to get them cleaned. One chair's covering was peeling so badly that I took it apart to recycle the metal and threw away the rest. It seems that we keep finding things to sell as we downsize.

Speaking of visiting Dad, yesterday as he was scheduled to see the surgeon. But LifePace didn't have a ride available for him. He had a shower earlier in the day and was in quite a bit of discomfort. The Physician Assistant (PA) came through and said that Dad had been placed on stronger pain medication than Tylenol, so he is now on narcotics. He is on a small dose but with the understanding that he will probably need more. The ladies say he won't hardly eat for them. Julia got him to eat more than half of his entree, some of the potatoes, and half of the pudding. He talked a lot of the time but he was hard to understand as usual. One thing he still does is pray with us when we pray. The TV in his room was on a local Christian station when we arrived, which was nice.

Charlotte visited with Dad again tonight. She was distressed with how Dad was. I told her we were troubled by it also. Alzheimer's disease and the fall are taking a toll on him. I want to be with him more, but there is so much that needs to be done. I will return tomorrow. I am afraid that Dad isn't going to make it much longer. I don't want him to remain in pain. I can't explain it, but God has given me a feeling of peace. Why is Dad experiencing this? I don't know.

But I know that Dad belongs to God, He has Dad in His hands. Dad's physical condition is at a place where I can't do it all for him. And I'm not able to take Mom to her brother's funeral, I have to rely on others. Maybe that is what I need to learn. My body isn't able to do all that I used to do. I have more aches and pains. I get tired more easily. However, I can do a lot. On Friday Dad is to see the surgeon so hopefully we will know more then about his condition.

There was a shooting at one of the doctor's office buildings of the St. Francis health system in Tulsa today. There is a change coming to America. I believe God is putting us in a place to prepare us for revival. Christians will be tested severely, I'm afraid. I want to be ready for what Jesus has for me to do.

Mom's brother passed away Sunday evening the same day that Mom and her sister were able to talk to him together on a call. And his kids all got to see him. One of Mom's sister's daughters, their niece, said that Mom's brother had prayed and given his life to God. He wanted his niece and then his son-in-law to pray that afternoon after many of the other family members left. Later that night he went to be with the Lord. Mom was heartbroken and Charlotte went to stay the night with her. The rest of us kids texted and talked to Mom off and on. Charlotte and Nick have acquired tickets for her and Mom to attend his service. I want to go with them, but need to be here for Dad. I talked to mom about it and she said that she understood. There is just a lot of tough stuff to deal with right now. I'm glad that I have God to get me through it all, as well as having Julia. Wow, what a blessing she has been to me! I pray that I am as much of a help to her as she is to me.

Chapter 10

Preparations For a Tough Decision

JUNE 2, 2022

THIS WAS A good day for me. Julia drove one of our granddaughters, Alyson, with her mom, Hayley, to Oklahoma City for Alyson's doctor's appointment. This gave me the day alone to spend time with God and to reflect on things. As far as Dad is concerned, it was as if God was leading me. I went to see Dad with the intent of talking to someone about his condition, prognosis, and potential outlook on what is best for him. I was able to confer with three of the therapists who have worked with Dad, who were taking a break together. They said that Dad hasn't responded well to therapy and resists the efforts of the therapists to get him up and going. They dressed him this morning to get him up but he seemed to be in so much pain that they put him back to bed and ordered an X-ray to check his hip. Later we hoped to find out if the hip was still in place. He is scheduled to see the surgeon tomorrow for a follow-up procedure to check his healing progress.

I was offered a plate of food from the cafeteria to eat with Dad, so I took it: ribs, baked beans, and broccoli salad. It was good. It took about forty-five minutes but I coaxed Dad to eat about half of his plate. He doesn't try to eat on his own. He has lost another 17 lbs since he has been in the facility. After the x-rays were taken and he had eaten, Dad went to sleep. I sat with him until I found out about the results of the X-rays. The X-rays didn't reveal much, not enough to tell if his hip was still in place. The surgeon should be able to tell us more tomorrow. So I read the Bible from the book of Colossians with Dad before he went to sleep.

Earlier in the morning, I had gotten up early to pray and read the Bible as usual, but today was more urgent. I prayed as I drove the 30 minutes to see Dad. I also prayed on the way home and God touched my heart in a special way leaving me with comfort and peace. In the past, I would worry about these things and struggle to sleep as I would torment myself over things. The issue with Julia's dad seems to be coming to an end which will be a huge relief. The other house should sell fairly easily which will be another huge burden lifted. Many of our financial needs will be met by selling the house in town. I feel that this summer is going to be a pivotal time in our lives. It will be nice to only have to worry about caring for Dad and not these other things.

Today, as I sit and reflect on the last few years of our lives, all of it is such an eye-opening picture of how God has provided for us in so many ways. It is obvious that He urged or prodded us into some ways we would preferred to not have taken. It is in those times that He revealed Himself to us so beautifully and without those hard circumstances, we wouldn't have been able to experience God as we have. In Sunday School class we are studying the Upper room discourse that Jesus had with his disciples. In the book of John, chapters 14 to 16, Jesus told his disciples that they would have difficulties but to not be discouraged by these trials. It is through these trials that God will be able to lead them to heights they can't imagine. I have learned that each of us has a role to play in the life we have been given. It's our choice to allow God to direct us so we can experience what He has for us. We can choose to be halfhearted followers. Or we can choose to resist Him completely. It's up to us. Jesus chose to fully follow the path laid out by His Father thereby pointing us to the path of a life with God that He intended us to have and that He desires to have with us. We have to surrender to Him as Jesus submitted to His Father.

An example for me is the relationship that Julia and I have. My dream has been to have a great marriage that will enable Julia and me to both be all that God wants us to be. Well, to have that both of us have to fully surrender to God individually. Through various events, we have both been challenged to pursue God in our unique ways. Our pursuits have produced a bond between us that we would not have been able to create through our own efforts. Yesterday was an example of that: Julia was able to share in our granddaughter's health journey and I was able to spend time working my way through meeting Dad's needs and dealing with my feelings, desires, emotions, etc. It was a comfort to see Dad resting instead of being as uncomfortable as he had been on many previous days. It was as if God were sending me a message that Dad would be OK. I have to let go and allow others to be a part of his life journey at this point. I will still be a huge part, but I don't have to carry the burden alone as I often think I have to do.

This all happened on Thursday, today is Friday. We were going to run our garage sale today, but we decided last night to wait until Saturday. We are both tired and Dad's doctor appointment is this morning. Julia would have to work the garage sale alone on Friday as I will be at the doctor with Dad, instead we will both go. It is forecasted to rain on Saturday, but that has been moved to the evening hours and Sunday. That will help. It is as if the weather is being tailor-made for our schedule.

By the way, our granddaughter, Alyson, has a diagnosis and that should be helpful. Now she has some answers, hopefully, proper treatment will help her overcome her struggles. It took over four hours at the doctor, but if she gets better it will be worth it. What a great day!!

June 3, 2022

We met Dad at the surgeon's office for his appointment. LifePace provided transportation. Dad was obviously in pain. He was dressed in one of his snap shirts, jeans, and socks. We got him on the bed for the X-rays but it hurt Dad a lot. Moving from the X-ray room to the exam room to meet the doctor was rough. The X-rays revealed the hardware used to repair Dad's broken hip had come loose. It seems Dad's bones are too soft to hold the screws necessary to repair his hip. This is probably what is causing his pain.

A second surgery is needed. After talking with the surgeon, we decided to go with the removal of the hardware and let Dad's bones heal as they will, and he will not walk again. Dad was moaning the whole time we were there. Arrangements were made for us to immediately take Dad to the hospital for his pre-op appointment right away. Since the surgeon's office and the hospital were connected, we could take Dad in his wheelchair.

Still, it was quite a ways to the hospital pushing Dad in the wheelchair. He kept sliding down in the chair and his feet were dragging on the floor. I tried pulling him backwards but his feet kept dragging and that wouldn't work. I prayed and we tried readjusting Dad. I lifted him and Julia pushed the wheelchair under him, which sat him up straighter. We positioned both of his feet on one of the footrests. He still moaned a little but we were able to push him much better.

After a bit Dad seemed to be more comfortable and his moaning subsided. When we got to the main entrance and checked in, Dad seemed to be fine. It seems that sliding down and sitting low in the chair caused the pain but sitting up straight was more comfortable. When we were able to get in the room for his pre-op procedure he was much better. The next challenge was drawing blood. Dad was dehydrated and his veins wouldn't rise much. After five or six attempts, success! Dad tolerated this for the most part.

Preparations For a Tough Decision

Then we had quite a wait for Dad's ride to arrive. But Dad was fine. The surgery is scheduled for Monday and we are glad to have it done. The driver to take Dad back to the skilled nursing facility was one of the young men who often took Dad to the ADHC center. He always took extra time to get Dad comfortable before transporting him. It was nice to see him. Dad's legs were getting red and indicated mottling from sitting in the wheelchair. His legs looked better after he was in bed for a while.

Throughout the day's events, two different people mentioned hospice care for Dad. He wouldn't have to move for therapy and the pain management is more aggressive as at this point addiction isn't a concern. This may be an option we pursue if the surgery doesn't relieve his pain.

This has been quite a day with lots of emotions and discussions. I even approached one of the nurses who hasn't been involved with Dad as far as I know and asked for her input about hospice care. Her observations were very informative. This discussion continued later with my siblings and Mom. There are tough things to consider and decide. Looking back, the last couple of days prepared me for what is to come. Again, God is so good!

Julia and I had a great prayer time together when we got home. It was very helpful for me. I have peace but still struggle with seeing Dad as he is. As I have stated, this isn't what I wanted for him. But God is in control and He is with Dad and us. Dad isn't alone.

June 4, 2022 — Saturday

Yesterday Julia and I had dinner with Charlotte before visiting with Dad. At this time, our emotions were all over the place. Our visit was good. I struggle with the fact that Dad is in this condition. I didn't want things to go this way. I feel like I have failed Dad. More and more, I feel like God wants me to learn that I am not in control and to let Him take care or use others to help me. Even knowing this, I struggle with guilt even though I know Dad is in God's hands.

I feel bad that Dad doesn't do as well with the staff, but performs better when we are there. He eats more and cooperates more with such things as taking medicine, being changed, etc. We helped a lot more tonight. I wasn't sure if I should be doing as much as I did and didn't want to get the staff in trouble. I know it is a struggle to change Dad as he isn't cooperative and it does hurt him, and none of us want to hurt him. So when we are there I make sure to offer to help as much as I can. I fed him as much of the dinner as he would eat.

He has a bed sore on his lower back a the top of his crack, it looks horrible and smells bad. His left heel looks as if a sore may be developing. We showed it to the nurse's aid who put a barrier spray and padded boot on it. Hopefully, the spot won't break as it is just a blister at this time. Julia looked up some stuff about the sores and read it to me on the way home. Hopefully, Dad doesn't get any more of these. I didn't realize that the sores can begin in just hours. With Dad not wanting to move off of his right side and it is difficult to find a position that doesn't cause him any pain, so he stays in the same position for extended times to keep his discomfort down. Tonight I helped to secure him more on his left side for the night and helped with his evening medications. But he will probably shift himself to the other side as he often does.

I also fed him. When the Certified Nursing Assistance (CNA) came in she wanted to know what I did to get him to eat. A little later the medical technician showed me a way to hold his head comfortably in a position that makes it easier for him to swallow. That helped when I fed him later. Instinctively I believe Dad knows who we are and he is familiar with us, which may be one of the reasons he will eat for us. He has lost so much of his cognitive ability since the fall.

Preparations For a Tough Decision

Part of my guilt I feel is that I should be there more often to help him more. But we have so many other things to do, it is difficult. We had our garage sale on Saturday, but didn't sell much. I had brought down quite a bit of stuff that had been stored for many years. The day was slow. We decided this would be the last day to try to sell anything so we dropped off some clothes for Goodwill. We will deal with the other stuff later.

Tomorrow, my sister, Tina and her husband Andy, and another sister Charlotte and her husband Nick, are coming to visit Dad. Mom and Gary may come. I don't think Dad will last long. The anesthesia needed for surgery isn't great for dementia patients. So there is no telling how this surgery will affect him.

Chapter 11

Second Surgery

JUNE 5, 2022 — SUNDAY

TINA, ANDY, AND Charlotte visited Dad with us. Tina spent time alone with Dad. Charlotte and I have already had private conversations with Dad. We aren't sure what he understands but we feel it is important to let him know we love him and that everything is OK between us. He is free to go on to Heaven if the Lord calls him. He is in a miserable state and none of us want him to hang on account of us feeling that we aren't ready for him to go. This is so tough!

Jason and one of our grandsons, Allen, took the dresser from our house in town and we put it in Jason's room. They also helped me move the treadmill and put Dad's mattress upstairs. These things had been in the house we are selling. Julia and I were tired and fussed some, enough that we needed to spend some time apologizing and making things right later that day. The strain can get to you sometimes. Jason's shoulders were hurting him and he had a lot of things that he was trying to get done. So I was trying to hurry for Jason's sake but Julia wanted me to have Jason and Allen help with a couple of other things while they were there. But I wasn't up to moving them. Anyway, Julia and I made up and things are OK. This happens now and then. But God sees us through.

June 6, 2022—Monday

Dad had surgery to remove the hardware from his hip. During the process the Operating Room (OR) team had one of the doctors here check Dad's sore on his backside, resulting in treatment while he was in the OR where the sore was trimmed and cleaned. It was bad. Today was the first time I got a look at Dad's sore since the doctor at the skilled nursing center took a look at it. That feeling of guilt that I have let Dad down resurfaced. My intent is to get Dad to a place closer to home so we can check on him more. He was in such pain that it seemed cruel to move him, but now we have another issue to address.

Tina and Charlotte were here today also. This morning, before Dad was taken for surgery we wiped him with the sanitizing pads that were provided and did all we could to get fluids down him before 11:30 am when he was supposed to stop ingesting anything. He did eat a spoon of pudding with Tylenol at that time. LifePace transported him to St. Francis in a wheelchair transport for surgery to remove the rods and pins that had been used to fix his broken hip. I rode with Dad. The ride showed up early, but that worked out well. St. Francis staff took him right in and began the preliminary procedures. Then we did have to wait a bit, but Dad wasn't in pain. We will have to wait and see how things go after he starts coming around tomorrow. I pray that God can guide us to the proper treatment for Dad from this point.

Later after the surgery, we are at St. Francis South in a Level 2 ICU unit. Dad went in for surgery at 4:00 pm and is still fairly well out of it. You can tell his leg is not in its natural place but he didn't seem to hurt as much when he was shifted to the side slightly to get him off of the sore. It did hurt. Maybe the anesthesia is still affecting him. We tried to get some Tylenol with applesauce down him, but he wouldn't swallow, even with a little water. The nurse had to suction everything from his mouth, clean, and lubricate inside his mouth. The risk is that the foodstuff would go into his lungs and cause another issue. Hopefully, tomorrow he will be able to eat. At least now he isn't in as much pain.

It has been a long day. I am tired. Tina spent the night at the house with Julia so she didn't have to drive home in the dark. Julia and Tina will be back tomorrow for a while. I will be getting to bed in the room with Dad soon to sleep as well as I can in the hospital. This is never an enjoyable thing.

June 7, 2022—The day after surgery

We were up and going at 4:30 this morning. The anesthesia has worn off and Dad seemed to feel the pain. The nurse got Dad started on morphine. He has had pain medication on a regular schedule today. The surgeon stopped by to check on him. Also, the hospital doctor, infectious disease doctor, Physical Therapist, and Speech Pathologist stopped by. The Speech Pathologist determined that Dad wasn't swallowing well enough to eat and drink. Dad's sore on his backside has created a potential for infection and he has a low-grade fever occasionally. When we first saw him yesterday morning, he was clammy and sweaty. So I am not surprised. The Physical Therapist couldn't even get Dad to sit on the side of the bed so she said she would be back in a couple of days. They consistently shift him to keep pressure off of one point too long. We don't want any more sores.

Speaking of sores, a nurse who specializes in wounds like this came to treat and clean Dad's sore. She was VERY informative. Since Dad's sore was so deep, it had been festering for quite a while, possibly months. I do remember times in the last few months when I had to clean Dad and he acted like it hurt to clean at the upper portion of the crack on his backside but I couldn't find a reason why he had pain. This may have been the cause. She said unless you know what to look for you won't know about what is going on under the skin until the skin breaks and you have a good sized legion like Dad has.

The spots on his heels likely happened at the skilled nursing center as he kept pressing his left heel into the mattress. The last couple of years for some reason, his feet have been pressing together. Often, I would need to pry his feet apart to dress him. As far as the sore on his behind, I assumed that we moved him from the wheelchair to the recliner, to the table, had him standing to dress him, to put him to bed was enough movement to prevent sores. But it may have not been.

Her explanation about these sores helped me feel better. I was feeling guilty that the Dad had been neglected by all of us who had been caring for him and causing the soreness. Knowing that a sore of this depth couldn't have developed in the time since he broke his hip helps to relieve some of the guilt I was feeling. I did ask Dad's case manager if there was the possibility of a facility closer to home for Dad when he gets out of the hospital so I could be more involved in his treatment and care. While he was in the facility in south Tulsa, which is thirty minutes away, I wasn't able to be with Dad as much as I wanted.

Dad wasn't eating very much at the skilled nursing facility for the workers there. He eats better for me. I was discouraged this morning, but I feel much better this evening. After the sore was cleaned, Dad didn't seem to have as much pain. I believe he gets tired of lying so much and wants to go home. Still, I'm not sure that can happen soon, if at all, but we will see.

I talked to Dad's case manager at LifePace asking if they will let us know if hospice care was a possibility as the pain management is different and more aggressive. Dad's case manager said they were meeting to discuss cases later and would discuss Dad's case at the meeting. Then she will get back to me. It has been a long day and I am tired but feeling more hopeful. God is good!!!

The infection doctor stopped by later in the day to discuss treatment of Dad's bedsore. To treat the lesion appropriately, Dad will need 6 weeks of antibiotics in a Long Term Acute Care Hospital, or LTACH, when he is stabilized here. The sore is more of a concern to the doctors than his hip is at this point. It hurts my heart that this happened to him. We aren't sure when the sore began, maybe more aggressive treatment could have been taken but Dad wasn't able to understand what needed to be done to treat him. He wouldn't eat for others very often, he wouldn't stay in positions in which he was placed, resisted efforts of Physical Therapists and others who were trying to help him get better or care for him.

Dad lost around twenty pounds since he broke his hip. I came when I could to help, but we had a lot of things to do. I know Dad preferred that I care for him. Hopefully, we will be able to get the house ready to sell soon also. We are afraid the market will fall sour soon and we don't want to miss that window to get the best deal we can. This all still breaks my heart and leaves me feeling guilty that I have let Dad down.

Then Gary sent a text that his pickup radiator connector broke. The radiator has to be replaced but I won't be able to fix it due to caring for Dad. Gary found a shop that would do it for him for a decent price. I usually fix these things for him and I am glad he found a way to get it fixed economically.

June 9, 2022—Friday — A pivotal day

God works in many ways, today is no exception. Dad is more aware of things today. He can swallow and has been given the OK to begin eating, but when I try to get him to eat today he knocks my hand away. He hasn't done that to me very often and usually, he will do things when I ask. From what they told me he has had a high sodium content in his system which can cause confusion and reduced cognitive ability.

The last two weeks or so he hasn't been eating or drinking enough, therefore dehydration allows the sodium levels to increase. Since the surgery he has been given some nutrition through his IV, leveling his sodium level.

Now his sodium levels are more stable, he can give me indications of what he wants. He doesn't act like anything hurts, he expresses more of an aggravated growl because he doesn't want to be disturbed. I get the feeling he is ready to give up and that is what he is trying to tell me. He and I had this conversation years ago when we realized that he had Alzheimer's disease and before he wasn't able to make these decisions for himself, he wanted me to make those for him. Then he signed the Living Will and Do Not Resuscitate (DNR) to express those desires. Now that the time seems to be approaching, I don't know that I want to make that decision.

Later that day, the hospice doctor stopped by. He had stopped by a couple of times since Dad's surgery and I always felt better after talking with him. This time he came in while one of the nurses was tending to Dad and sat down with me. As we talked about Dad, at one point he mentioned that there are times that we have to make hard decisions in these situations. I knew that this moment would come at some point and this visit by the doctor was a gift from God.

In the back of my mind, I think I knew it was time but I didn't want to accept that. When the doctor visited me and suggested it may be time, that took a load off my shoulders!! I almost felt that he was God's way of giving me permission to let Dad go. I was heartbroken and broke down in tears but I knew this was the time. I had prayed many times that Dad would quietly go into his sleep one night so I wouldn't have to face this moment, but God had other plans. I finally told the doctor and the nurse that I was ready, but wanted to visit with my family first. I later learned that the doctor actually started Dad on comfort care the first time I said that I was ready to start Dad on hospice because Dad needed the extra pain medicine to be comfortable.

After a discussion with my brother, sisters, Mom, and dad's sister, they all agreed with the decision to start Dad on hospice care. Especially after the description of all that the treatment on Dad's backside will involve I know that Dad will prefer not to go through that ordeal. Besides he was ready to go to heaven. We aren't sure what to expect, so we take one day at a time.

Charlotte and Mom are heading to Wyoming for Mom's brother's funeral so Charlotte is struggling with being gone and worrying that Mom will feel guilty that she is keeping Charlotte from being here with Dad. Mom and I had a good talk on the phone when she settled in at my cousin's in Powell, Wyoming. It won't surprise me that Dad will still be here when Charlotte returns from the funeral with Mom.

June 10, 2022

Dad is still hanging in there. He hasn't moved and at this point moving him disturbs him so I don't see any reason to move him. He gets morphine every two hours so he doesn't moan or act like anything is hurting him. He responded when I talked to him and rubbed his head. His vital signs are still good, better than I thought they would be this morning.

I put a post on social media to let as many people as I could know about putting Dad on hospice care. I talked to his sister yesterday and prayed with her over the phone before the final decision was made. I also let Dad's primary care doctor know. The hospital chaplain stopped by to visit and pray with me. Friends came by last night which helped.

My mind is all over the place. I keep thinking about what I should say at his service, should we have it at Muse, should we cremate him and bury his ashes, or have a traditional burial? So many options. Will we be able to give him a good service? Going to Muse, which is 4 hours from Tulsa, for the service will prevent a lot of the people we know from being able to attend. Am I being selfish in any way? Do my siblings have desires or ideas but don't want to say anything and leave the decisions up to me? I've started putting together the pictures that I have of Dad for a slide show. If we go to Muse I don't know if they have a projector for a slide show.

I still have raw emotions but feel at peace. Tina, Mishelle, and Mishelle's son, Steven, are coming up today. Her son may bring his kids. I plan to give Dad's prison jacket to Steven if he wants it, since he now works as a prison guard, following in Dad's footsteps as Dad served as a guard for several years. Well, I better get something to eat.

June 12, 2022

It is Sunday morning. I am home with Julia. Tina and Mishelle stayed with Dad Friday and Saturday nights. Julia and I moved a bunch of things from the other house, taking two pickup loads to a charity in town. They acted excited to get the items. We had a pickup load to take to the house where we were moving. Julia is hoping that one of her newfound cousins will be able to take the school stuff to her daughter so someone can use it. Then I need to clean out the shop and two sheds. With one more good day of moving and cleaning, we should have the house ready to sell.

Dad is still hanging in there. He does spend quite a bit of time looking around, moving now and then, and at times reacting to something that happens in the room. It seems at times he is snickering when someone laughs or does something funny. The morphine drip is now on a three. The nurse started it on one and she said it goes to ten. The goal is to give him what he needs to be comfortable. If he isn't stable he will stay at the hospital. If he becomes stable then he will be able to go to a hospice house if a room becomes available in one of the local end of life care facilities. He won't have the IV hydration at the hospice house so all he will have is what he can take orally. We just don't want him to be in pain.

Julia suggested that Dad doesn't want to go, especially with family around him. She may be right. Dad enjoyed having his family around. He may be in a state of mind that he isn't able to realize the poor condition of his body since he is medicated and he will be in a lot of pain if the medication

Second Surgery

is stopped. He doesn't want to live in this state but he may not realize the state in which he is. Alzheimer's disease is cruel. I greatly appreciate my sisters staying with Dad to allow me to be with Julia doing what we need to get done. Hopefully, we can get the house ready to sell while houses are still selling well. This trend can't last forever.

Mom's brother's funeral wasn't as expected. Mom and her sister were very disappointed and hurt. They didn't get much attention as it seemed that the attention was on his wife's family. Mom, Charlotte, and Mom's sister sat in a back corner but not with family from what I understood. The service was short with a couple of songs and a couple of readings but I don't believe there was any scripture read, preaching, or much prayer. The consolation is that Mom's brother made his peace with God and told Mom that he would see her in a better place. One of Mom's nieces confirmed that Uncle Jimmy had given his heart to God. That helps. It also helps that Mom, Charlotte, and Mom's sister are staying with Mom's niece and getting to spend time with her and Mom's sister. I don't know if they have seen any of the other nieces or been able to spend time with any of Mom's brother's kids. We have the same issue with Julia's dad and brother. It's sad that families have these divisions.

Gary's truck has a broken radiator. He isn't able to get it fixed until Friday. With Dad's condition and all we need to get done, I am not able to get over to fix it for him. I don't know if he could come to spend much time with Dad if he had a way. Charlotte's husband will bring him but Gary doesn't want to as it is painful. He has a difficult time being able to sit unless it happens to be a certain kind of chair due to his back issues. The chairs at the rehab facility were hard. There isn't anything comfortable at the hospital either. So I can understand, that his health has gotten to the point that he is miserable all the time. Losing weight would solve a lot of his problems. His dilemma is a struggle for most of us.

JUNE 13, 2022

I texted our pastor to let him know that no one from church has called or visited us since Dad has been in the hospital. The church staff had sent us a card wishing Dad well when he first went into the hospital after his fall. But nothing since then. Soon, we had a visit from our pastor's dad, then a couple from our Sunday School class later in the day. Our grandson, Allen, stopped by while the pastor's dad was here. Later our grandson, Jason, and his wife Maci, came by to visit. So the day was busy with visitors, which was nice. I didn't mean to upset our pastor but I feel as pastors they need to know we hadn't had any interaction from our church, especially since we have been in the church so long and this is a major life event for us. Maybe I am wrong but people need to know that your church family cares in situations like this.

Dad's nurse from LifePace, called me today. She has been on vacation. I updated her on where we are. The case worker emailed and I gave her an update. Also, Dad's sister called for an update. She said that she is doing OK She didn't seem to realize that we had already started Dad on Hospice care. I let her know it won't be too long. She said that she was OK but she didn't sound too much like it. Her daughter is facing some health issues and a divorce. Poor girl feels so defeated. Dad's sister has a lot going on in her life also.

Mom and Charlotte will be home from Wyoming later tonight. Charlotte will be coming to see Dad in the morning. I'm not sure that Mom will come with her, but it wouldn't surprise me if she did. I hope Dad's appearance isn't too much of a shock to them as he isn't very responsive at this time.

Hopefully, Dad won't tarry long. He may not want to go but with the dementia caused by the Alzheimer's disease, his mind isn't able to comprehend the gravity of his situation. Julia feels that he is hanging on especially as he hears the voices of his family. His vital signs stay strong.

Second Surgery

JUNE 15, 2022

A lot has happened. Yesterday morning, the hospice nurse and floor nurse both said that they felt that Dad was definitely down to his last days, probably his last hours. I sent a message to my siblings to that effect. They all came within hours. Tina and Andy came first. Charlotte went to work to tend to a couple of things so she would be free for the rest of the week if needed. Mishelle came later with her husband, Alan, and two boys. Charlotte's husband, Nick, brought Mom and Gary. Julia had scheduled to meet with two of her cousins to work on cleaning the house in town, but she came later. It was nice to have some help with our house.

Anyway, all of Dad's immediate family was here. We all spent time with him: as a whole group, the seven consisting of Mom and the five kids of Mom and Dad, then various groups through the evening. We spent time remembering good times and sharing memories. We as a group told Dad that we were ready for him to go and that he was free to go. We believe it is important to let a loved one know that you are ready for them to go. We prayed together also. We believe that Dad's spirit left him at this point.

During the night Gary and Nick, went to Charlotte and Nick's house to sleep. Andy, Mishelle, Alan, and Charlotte slept in their cars. Mom and Tina slept in the room with Dad. Mishelle's boys went home. Julia and I stayed in the waiting room. I arranged a chair close to the round large table in the middle of the waiting room putting my legs on the table and my head on the arm of the chair with my body in the chair to lie down. After a while one of the nurses brought out one of the couches that lay into a bed out to the waiting area with a pillow and blanket for me to sleep. I was appreciative and felt fussed over more than necessary. I eventually fell asleep until 5:00 am.

I awoke to see Julia sleeping on two chairs she had pulled together to make a bed of sorts in which she was scrunched in so she could fit. I felt bad that she had to do that but I had a place to stretch out. I finally convinced her to lie on the bed I had been given so she could stretch out and rest for a couple of hours. The couch had to be returned to the room before the day shift at 7:00 am. All of us kids wanted to be close to Dad at this point.

Dad still hung in there with little change. His morphine level was at an eight to start the day, then was increased to nine later. His Tylenol drip continued. His vital signs didn't change much. We again shared memories and discussed future arrangements for Dad's service so that we could ponder on them until we needed to sit down and make the final decisions. Later in the day, the nurse increased Dad's morphine to level ten. They gave Dad a frontal sponge bath and changed his gown. The last four nurse shifts have consisted of two nurses with the same name, one on the day shift who was pregnant and the other on the night shift was not pregnant. Dad's vitals were indicating more change in his body's condition. He was putting out very little urine, his heart rate was trending over 100 and his breathing was becoming shallow.

Chapter 12

The Final Days

June 15, 2022 — Day 7 on Hospice

DAD IS STILL hanging on. We aren't sure what is keeping him. There hasn't been much change in the last three or four days. His heart rate will increase a little but never trend over 100. His oxygen level is rarely below 90. His breathing rate has been around 15 breaths per minute most of the day. When his bandage was changed around 7:00 pm his heart rate rose to 120 and his oxygen level fell to the 70s and 80s. His breathing rate increased to 25 or so and you could hear fluids in his lungs. But after three hours his numbers all leveled back about the same as they were before moving him and his lungs sounded clear. Morphine level is on thirteen with Tylenol this morning. He has had a low fever all day. Normally the maximum morphine level is ten. Since Dad is still here the decision was made by his doctors to raise his morphine level. I'm not sure why.

Julia went home at midday to rest and check on Sam, her dog. She ended up staying at home the rest of the day and night. Tina and her husband stayed at the hospital all day and night. Charlotte stayed all day but went home around 10:30 pm. Mishelle and Alan stayed home as nothing was happening. Mom and Gary stayed most of the day until dinnertime. Nick had gone home the night before, then he went to school for a while.

He returned around lunchtime and stayed until dinnertime when he took Mom and Gary home. So Tina, Andy, and I are the ones who stayed for the night on Wednesday.

We were hoping that by shifting to change his bandage, maybe things would start to progress toward Dad's passing. But Dad doesn't seem to want to go. Most of us are convinced that yesterday when we were all here and praying together, Dad's spirit left at that time and just his body is lying here refusing to submit to death. Many times it was expressed that Dad was always one to do things his way and always quite the stubborn one. His eyes don't have any expression and he doesn't react to touch unless for a reflective grasp when you hold his hand. He didn't try to resist being moved when he was changed or repositioned during the day. His hands don't seem as swollen as they were and his urine output has increased. It is just a waiting game at this time. None of us have any idea why it is taking this long. This is the seventh day since hospice was started. We know we will see him again in Heaven.

One of the nurses brought out one of the couches from one of the other rooms for me to sleep on Tuesday night and said that she would do it again for tonight. It is 11:30 so I hope that she will bring it soon. My siblings are making it their goal that I don't stay alone at the hospital with Dad again. I pray that Dad goes soon. We are all exhausted. And he is ready to go.

June 16, 2022 — Day 8 on hospice

I went home for the night to get some rest. Charlotte, Tina, and Andy stayed the night at the hospital. Not much changed during the night. It was nice for me to get to sleep in my bed. The next morning, Tina and Andy went home fairly early. Charlotte slept at the hospital until Julia and I arrived around 9:30. We all three went downstairs so Charlotte could eat some breakfast. Julia ate as well. I had already eaten a large breakfast at home.

The Final Days

June 17, 2022 — Day 9 on hospice

After Charlotte left, the nurses came in to bathe Dad and change his bedding and bandage. Julia and I left the room while they took care of Dad. Not long after this Dad's heart rate and oxygen started to drop. Around 2:00 pm his heart rate increased to compensate for the low oxygen level that had dipped into the sixties. His respiration rate was fifteen to twenty. His heart rate was 115 or so. At 2:45 things leveled out with his heart rate at 105 and his oxygen was in the low 60s or high 50s. All in all his vitals indicate that his body is giving out. He probably won't be able to maintain long at that rate.

Two hours later everything leveled out again. His heart rate remained between 80 and 100 and his oxygen was in the 50s and 60s for a while. But later his oxygen leveled off in the 60s and 70s, sometimes dipping into the 80s. There is no telling how long this will continue.

All three girls decided to return to the hospital when I first informed them that his vital signs dropped. So I decided to come home again for the night. Charlotte also returned home. Mishelle and Alan left for the hospital after Alan got off work so they got to the hospital a little late. Two of our friends came up to visit again which was nice.

June 18, 2022 — Day 10 on hospice

Tina, Mishelle, and their husbands stayed with Dad last night. Tina and Andy slept in the room, Mishelle and Allen slept in their SUV on a bed in the back of the vehicle.

Julia and I spent the morning getting the sheds and backyard of the house in town cleaned. All we have left to move now are the things in the garage. We were able to get back to the hospital by 2:00 or so. We want to do some cleaning and touching up around the house before we put it up for sale. We planned to sell it ourselves at first but now we are leaning toward having a Realtor sell it for us. Still, we have some work before putting it on the market. The struggle has been dealing with this and Dad's situation. Also, I have someone teaching my Sunday School class at church in the morning so the class can meet even though Julia and I won't be there. I don't know why I didn't think of that last week when I canceled class.

Tina and Andy left for home around 3:00. Mishelle and Allen left at 5:00 to go home, visiting their son on the way. My siblings all agree that this has been a bonding experience that has brought us closer. God brings something good comes out of adversity.

Dad's numbers today have been fairly consistent. His heart rate has been in the 80s for the most part, his oxygen level has been anywhere from 60s to 80s, and his respiration rate has been in the upper 20s. Later in the day, Dad was making a noise quite often as he took a breath. Also, I don't know if I have mentioned that Dad has been given some additional medicine to reduce the fluid buildup in his lungs. His morphine is on level fourteen and seems comfortable there. We are wondering if Dad is waiting for Father's Day to pass. His mom passed on Mother's Day in 1989.

Anyway, I am at the hospital alone with Dad as Julia went home to take care of Sam. She was torn as she wanted to be with me. If Dad passes in the night she or Jason will have to come get me. I don't think he will be gone during the night but he may surprise all of us, according to Andy as he reminded us that Dad does things his way. Mom and Gary haven't returned as Gary's truck isn't out of the shop yet with the new radiator. The garage couldn't get to it. It will hopefully be done on Monday.

When Dad does pass, our plan is for each of us to return home for a couple of days before we meet with the funeral home director to make arrangements. Then we can get together again to decide on plans for Dad's service, go through his things, and divide up what he has as keepsakes. He doesn't have much. After we take care of all of his end-of-life expenses then whatever is left of his finances will be divided between mom and the kids.

That is the way Dad wanted things to go. I'm glad I had him write it down, now we knew what he wanted. This was a blessing.

Next weekend is when our grandson and his wife's, Jason and Maci, have their wedding reception on Saturday. Charlotte will probably be the only one of my siblings who may attend. Mom may come with us. Gary more that likely won't be able to make it, so Julia and I may need to go get Mom to spend the night with us so she can attend. Hopefully, Dad will have passed on by then. Whatever the reason Dad is taking so long, God is in control. All of this has been a learning process for us. But I wouldn't give anything for all that God has done in my life in caring for Dad. God has promised that He will always be with us and hasn't let me down.

June 18, 2022, 11:30 pm—On the Eve of Father's Day.

Dad completed his journey on this earth thirty minutes before Father's Day. His heart rate increased and the nurse increased his morphine level to fifteen. He also received some medicine to decrease the fluid in his lungs. His heart rate at one point increased to 132, then dropped to 110 or so and stayed there. So I decided to lie down and go to sleep. I laid out some blankets on the couch in the room and wrapped them around me. But within five minutes Dad's heart rate was in the 60s.

I felt something was different but didn't realize until later, that Dad had stopped breathing. So I got up to be with him, pray, and say goodbye. His heart dropped to the 30s for a few beats, then stopped. A couple of seconds later there were a few more heartbeats, then nothing again. About then the nurse came in, and alarms started going off. In a bit, she confirmed that Dad was gone.

For a while earlier this evening before I decided to go to sleep, Dad's eyes were open. I talked to him, played some gospel music, and listened to my Bible lessons as I sat in the chair beside him. It was just the two of us. There was a sweet calmness and spirit present. Maybe he wanted it to be just the two of us. So many times he would surprise us by hanging on when it seemed there was no way for him to make it, but he did. I thought this time could be the same thing. But this is the first time that I saw his heart rate increase to 130. The nurse pointed out that his heart line on the monitor indicated irregular activity. So, he finally gave up, thirty minutes before Father's Day. I called Julia who came with Jason to get me. After Dad was taken by the funeral home, we went home.

JUNE 21, 2022

We met with the funeral home director today, three days after Dad passed. We scheduled Dad's service for July 8th due to varying issues, primarily family schedules. We decided to have Dad cremated, so we didn't need to hurry. By the time he spent ten days in hospice and not eating for over a month, his body was down to skin and bones. With the condition of his body, there is no way to have an open casket so we decided to have his body cremated. This brought the cost of his service down significantly and simplified the whole process. I struggled at one time with cremation but am okay with it now as are the rest of the family members.

I will present most of Dad's service with input from my siblings. Charlotte is working on the music. I am putting together a rough draft of the slide show and Nick will provide the finishing touches. We decided to use the chapel at the funeral home as our church is redoing the floor. We all provided input and I believe all are satisfied with how things are planned. Since Dad has been cremated, we have a couple of weeks to get things together which will help. I was struggling with needing to hurry to prepare for the service and having things ready in a few days but that was solved when we decided for cremation and waiting a few more days to have

The Final Days

the service. Having more time is a great relief. But it will be an even greater relief to have it all done. I want to do right by Dad.

JUNE 23, 2022

Yesterday, we worked getting the house in town ready to sell. There is a lot involved in getting this done. We still had Christmas items in the attic to move and there were a lot of touch-up items to complete: painting the bathroom ceiling, fixing a leaky faucet, floor tiles in the bathroom needed to be replaced, mowing and trimming, cleaning, switching microwaves even though the house we live in has a newer microwave, but we liked the one from the other house better, things like that. It almost seems to be endless. There always seemed to be one more thing to do.....

I become emotional at times going through the house remembering that this is the last home that Dad had. I believe he enjoyed his time here. The Alzheimer's disease took a lot from him but we did all we could to make life pleasant as possible for him. I went next door to let one of the neighbors know the last events of Dad's life as well as Dad's service times. She said that Dad had told her that he appreciated us helping him. He had told me that at times also, but hearing it from her gave my spirit a lift. Even though I have grieved Dad's passing for a while there are still times that things affect me in ways I didn't anticipate.

Dad's sister called to check on things. She assumed that we would have had Dad's service by now. She doesn't anticipate coming for Dad's service. She has some family issues, and is having a tough time. I pray for her. She is carrying a heavy load.

Charlotte and Nick have secured a cabin for us to stay after we take Dad's ashes to be buried at the New Home Cemetery, where Dad wanted to be buried. After the service and burial of Dad's ashes, Mom, my siblings, and our spouses will spend the weekend together. The cabin is in Broken Bow

What I Learned From Dad

and we will use some of the leftover money from Dad's funeral fund to pay for it. This will be one last time we will be together on Dad. It is too bad he can't be with us, but he would approve of us getting together one last time in his honor. We will have other family events in which we will remember him, but this is one more time to be together to remember and be thankful for the good fight that Dad fought. Now he is in Heaven rejoicing!

Chapter 13

Life After Dad

July 20, 2022

I T H A S B E E N a while since I have added to this story. It has been a whirlwind of things since returning from Broken Bow. We had a good time at the cabin. I just took it easy and didn't do much. Julia and I just took a short drive alone Saturday evening, since that day was our anniversary. We drove to a couple of the campgrounds and some of the shops, which were closed at that time of the day. The campgrounds and town are much different from when we had come on camping trips when we were kids, but it was nice to remember the good times. We haven't done anything for our anniversary yet. We have been busy trying to get our house, yard, shop, and gym in order.

We also put our house in town on the market. We were offered $2500.00 more than we asked on the same day the house was listed. We took the offer. As part of the process, the appraisal was conducted yesterday but we haven't heard the results. The major problem will be if the appraisal indicates the value of the house is too low and the bank won't approve the buyers for enough money to cover the cost of their offer. So we pray that the appraisal is enough to cover the amount offered. I am worried about the state of the foundation. Hopefully, the fact that we have stabilized the house with piers should solve that issue. It is a nice house but we don't need two houses. We are settled in the other house and want to live there.

We greatly enjoyed our time at the cabin. It was so nice to reconnect with my siblings and Mom. We need each other now that Dad is gone. It was as if Dad were there as he always enjoyed taking trips like this. It was hot but we stayed inside most of the time, at least most of us did. Tina and her husband took more time looking around the town where we were staying. We watched a couple of movies in the theater room, played pool on the table that was in the cabin, spent time on the porch during the morning coolness, some sat in the hot tub that was set so it wouldn't heat the water and on Friday night Julia and Charlotte had a fire in the fire-pit as there were still coals from the people who stayed in the cabin before us, we worked together to cook meals; all the things we used to do as a family when we were children.

Being July, it was hot so a hot tub and a fire weren't the most attractive amenities of the cabin. Most of my siblings have done similar activities with our families after we started our own families. While at the cabin we went through a lot of the pictures and keepsakes that Dad had and each of us kept things to remember Dad. I believe he would have been greatly pleased with us taking this time together, especially since funds left from his burial fund were available to cover the cost. He would have called it a "family project", one of his many unique phrases.

I haven't mentioned anything about Dad's service. We had put his service off for a while due to the 4th of July holiday and that some of our family already had plans. We hoped that people would be able to attend with more time to make those arrangements. But it didn't seem that there were any more people than if we had had the service days sooner after Dad's passing. The other concern is that Charlotte and I needed some time to pull things together for our parts in the service. I was stressed when we met with the funeral director on Tuesday after Dad passed when we assumed that Dad's service would be on the following Friday or Saturday. I have been working on putting together a tribute to Dad for quite a while, but I didn't have a finished product at that time.

There were the pictures to finish organizing for the slide show so that Nick could put those in a video format for us. Charlotte was putting together the music for the prelude and conclusion as well as singing two songs herself. I needed to talk to our pastor's dad and our cousin, Scott, to see if they would take part in the service, with our pastor's dad reading the obituary and Scott preaching "clean up" after me and finishing up the service. One other item I added later was to ask our pastor if he would welcome the audience and offer the opening prayer. This later played into my tribute to Dad as father and son working together, supporting and caring for one another. Dad told me many stories about how he helped his Dad in his later work years as Dad was the youngest son still at home as his dad aged.

There was the Honor Guard from the Department of Corrections, my nephew, Steven, a prison guard like Dad had been for a large part of his life, was able to arrange. This provided such a great finish to Dad's service. It was awesome. I have the flag presented during the funeral service in a case.

I believe the service went well. We have had several compliments on the tribute for Dad. I've also heard from many people who stated that they wouldn't be able to do what Charlotte and I did in Dad's service. Again, I know God wanted me to do this and Charlotte felt the same about singing. I believe Dad would have been very proud.

Before Dad had progressed too far into his Alzheimer's disease I asked him to write down what he wanted to be included in his funeral service. When Dad finished, I stored away what he had written without looking at it until he had passed away. On the last page, he wrote that he wanted his kids to say something at his service and that he desired just a graveside service. Since I didn't look at what he wrote until later after he passed, seeing

What I Learned From Dad

what he had written was another confirmation to me about speaking at his service. I also found in another place that he had put together a set of documents and made notes about his life that provided the majority of what I needed for his tribute. Of course, I added my content. But God had been putting the pieces together for us all along.

I spoke for about forty-five minutes but didn't plan to take that long. The service was about one and a half hours long. So many of those who attended didn't come to talk to us at the end as they needed to get back to work, etc. We needed to hurry to church for lunch, so we could head to New Home cemetery. We hoped to be at the cemetery around 4:30 and ended up being about fifteen minutes late, but being late didn't turn out to be a problem. We appreciated Rejoice Church for providing lunch for us after the service.

The young man digging and closing the grave wasn't in a hurry. Andy had been involved in many burials in the city where he worked and was very helpful in communicating with him. Everyone who was going to attend arrived by 5:00. We were able to head to the cabin around 5:15 or so after Dad's ashes were buried between his mom, Mamaw, and his aunt, Aunt Ruby. Charlotte had a small box with things to bury with Dad. Mishelle and her husband had car trouble getting to the cabin and missed Dad's burial. But they live close enough to visit the grave as often as they like.

We are working on securing a headstone for Dad. We found a place that is reasonably priced. But they are slow to respond, as many businesses are today. We had discussed what we wanted on his headstone together at the cabin. I have contacted them and am waiting for a response. We plan to pay for that out of Dad's insurance from the state due to his work as a prison guard from which he retired. We will share the rest between Mom and my siblings. I will pay taxes out of the funds since I am the beneficiary. But I want to make the sharing as even as possible as I believe that is what Dad would like.

We finally have the initial death certificates, that are "pending" a cause of death. There will be updated death certificates with an actual cause of death when the medical examiner gets to Dad's case, which could be up to six months. The updated certificates will enable me to apply for Dad's death benefit from the state. The funeral home will use one of the certificates to apply for his burial insurance funds. Hopefully, all of this will come together soon. By the way, the closing on the house will be September 3rd or before if everything comes together, as we pray it does.

The last major thing we need to finalize is with Julia's Dad. I have felt that this summer was Dad's last one and he passed right after I was out of school. Being out of school allowed me to be with him in the hospital and not be concerned with how things were going at school.

I also feel that we will be finalizing with James this fall. I have borrowed funds a couple of times to be ready to meet for a settlement because our lawyer said a meeting was pending. But the meetings never materialized. Oh well, live and learn. Both times I sent the money back after a couple of months of hanging on to it. Frustrating!!!

With Dad passing we've had time to arrange the house. Most of the downstairs is ready but the upstairs needs a lot of arranging. There is also a lot to do outside and the shop needs organizing as I just stacked things in there. And the heat is on outside. We have had several days of 100-degree temperatures and more is to come. And Julia is on a short trip with her friend, Alisa, and her friend's mom so I hope that I can finish some of the things I need to have done. I was lazy today, but hopefully, tomorrow I will have some energy to get things done.

AUGUST 11, 2022

My cousin, one of Dad's sister's daughters died yesterday afternoon. Her passing hit me hard and I don't know why. I expected her to overcome her sickness and return home. Maybe it was my reluctance to accept that she may not get well. Anyway, she is in a better place. I feel for her family as they have lost their dad, mom, and now a sister in the last two years. Not to mention the loss of my dad, their uncle.

I have talked to Dad's sister, off and on. She says she struggles with being the last of her siblings now that Dad is gone. She says she cries a lot. Her daughter, a granddaughter that she adopted, and her girl help keep her grounded. Her son is living on her property but he keeps to himself most of the time.

We have made a lot of progress on settling into the house. I replaced the kitchen sink and faucet for Julia removing the cast iron sink with a stainless steel sink that is deeper. We cleaned the windows something that was needed. Julia is slowly getting things in the bedroom as she likes. I still need to organize the shed and clean up the gym. I hope to get that done before school starts.

We will pre-sign the closing documents on the house. The buyers will sign on August 19th. We also need to mow it again. We are taking the extra freezer to Mom and Gary. The one in the house is twenty years old but keeps going. But they would like the upright that we have and they can give their chest freezer to our nephew. Our nephew has moved down to Muse and started work at the prison in Hodgens. I hope that it is going well for him there.

Most mornings Julia goes to a neighbor's garden to help him and give him some company. I need to do better at going over to see him. He is quite lonely without his wife, who passed away a year or so ago.

I have gone to one meeting at school and will go to one on Monday unless my cousin's funeral lands on that day. The last of our granddaughters who is still in high school started back to school today also. She seems to be doing well.

Life After Dad

We took one of our other granddaughters to look at a car that she and her mom had found in Tulsa. It seemed to be in good shape, just needed to be cleaned and the tires balanced. She went back later with her other grandma to buy it. So she is set to go to Colorado for school.

AUGUST 20, 2022

We signed the closing documents to sell our house on August 11th, the first day of school for Owasso. The buyers are signing their portions on August 19th at 3:30 pm on Friday. This will put off the pay-off for us until the following Monday. Our Realtor confirmed for us that the buyers did sign the closing documents so the selling of the house is a done deal. It feels strange knowing that we no longer have that house. We hope the people enjoy it and are a good fit for the rest of the neighbors. We received an email from the electric company that the electricity has been taken over by the new owners.

We went to dinner with friends last night to celebrate. It was nice to see them. I will be going with some of these friends to a NASCAR race in late September. I have never been to a race so this will be an adventure. I am sure that Julia and her friend will find some trouble to get into. We will leave on Friday night and return on Sunday.

Also, my cousin's funeral will be next weekend on the 27th of August. This will be a hard one to handle, she was too young. Another cousin who died about two years ago, was younger than that. It's hard to lose loved ones. Also, the wife of Mom's brother who passed away, had also passed away. No details or information. Her passing was just a little over ten weeks after he had died.

Our oldest granddaughter had her second baby. She is a beautiful baby and we wish we could see her. Julia and I wished we could have taken a trip to see them before school started but there were too many things happening. The one thing we need are the deeds from Julia's dad and then the documents to end the lawsuits and put that behind us. The first trip we will probably take will be to California to see Julia's family. Maybe in October during fall break. Hopefully, by then all of these things will be done. Also, we will be debt-free which will be a first for us since our time in Alaska. Hopefully, we follow God's will in the future, we are curious what God has in store for us. For now we are enjoying the time together to relax before the school year is in full swing.

We are slowly getting the smaller things around the house done. There will always be things to do but the place has been neglected so there is a lot to do. One notable thing was to clean out the electric water heater of the master bedroom and it hadn't been cleaned since it was installed, over 10 years ago. Boy was it a mess!! It took quite a bit to get it done. I have new heating elements if either of these fails. I bought them because I broke one of the seals putting the old ones back.

SEPTEMBER 22, 2022

What does God want us to do? This question is my current struggle. Sometimes I feel as if I should retire from teaching and do something in the line of a ministry, I'm just not sure what. So I try to keep my mind and heart open to what comes along. Our finances are in good shape. So we are seeking God's leading and praying for direction. We do enjoy that we have some freedom without the responsibility of Dad but it seems strange also. And I miss him.

Poor Sam, Julia's dog is struggling with his hips. He has a difficult time getting up. But he sure enjoys going on walks with Julia and to the garden with her in the mornings. He had a coughing and vomiting fit during the night last night. Julia isn't sure how long he will be able to last. She doesn't want him to suffer but she doesn't want to take away life from him if he enjoys it. He has helped her through some tough times. I have never been an animal lover, but this dog is a God-send for her and I am grateful for what Sam has done for her. Anyway, it's time to get ready for school and the day.

Speaking of school, I still do my best to foster a Godly, positive spirit at school. I share scriptures and devotions with other Christians at school and have a prayer group that meets weekly. I pray with parents who are comfortable with me doing so. We are called to be a light to the world. I want to shine for Him in any way that I can.

SEPTEMBER 30, 2022

School is in full swing. This year has been hard getting started. There isn't enough time to do all that needs to be done. And when you think you have it all in control, something else gets added to the pile. There are so many kids with severe needs who come to us without some of their basic needs being met. This results in kids engaging in behaviors at school seeking attention. I believe children's brains are developed or wired differently due to the increasing use of screened devices. Kids don't do as much reading, physical playing, or even interacting with each other or adults as much as twenty years ago. Problem-solving and relationship-building skills in kids are lacking.

Social media creates and fosters an attitude of expressing emotions, feelings, and opinions without being face-to-face with the people who are affected by what we say. So a lot is said without thinking about the effect of the words said or learning how to navigate the tricky maze of human emotions and feelings we all have. Learning to foster relationships with people is how we build the intimacy that we crave. This intimacy is what makes life rich, rewarding, and fulfilling. The same goes for our relationship with God. The more He does for us and the more difficult circumstances He brings us through, the more we love and appreciate Him and His love for us.

I have had a few talks with God. At times I am not sure if I am in God's will. I don't want to quit teaching as I do like what I do and enjoy being at work, but so many of the demands take from my time and being able to do more of what I want to do. Maybe this is God's way of moving me or letting natural circumstances push me into making a move. I like being a productive part of school but with Dad gone, I am not required to focus on him. After Dad went to bed, I had to stay home which was convenient and provided time for schoolwork in the evenings. Now I don't want to spend my evenings doing schoolwork since I am free to go and do other things. So I am going to have to make some adjustments.

> "Lord, lead me into making the right decisions and staying in your will. I know I will have You no matter what I do. But I do want to be a light for You and if You have a particular path for me, lead my heart and mind in that way. Also, let Julia have peace and understanding for the same thing. Lord, I love You and want to please You in all the ways that I can."

NOVEMBER 3, 2022

I was having a tough time at the beginning of this year, but this week I have turned a corner. In my mind, it seemed that I wasn't going to be able to get all of my work done. I felt overwhelmed most days. I was having a hard time at the beginning of the year keeping up with paperwork because I didn't spend as much time in the evenings on schoolwork as I had when caring for Dad. Baseball season is almost over and I will want to be out in my gym since there will be no St. Louis Cardinal ballgames to watch. I almost have it ready with a little more cleaning to do. I am ready to start working on getting back into shape. I have put on some excess weight in the last three years.

November 14, 2022

Yesterday would have been Dad's 84th birthday, his first birthday since he passed away.

The other night Charlotte had a dream of our family, Mom and the 5 siblings, in a church service together. As we were there in church she could see Dad in another location but as a much younger man dancing exuberantly, even though he couldn't ever dance. None of us have any rhythm, a trait we inherited from Dad. Anyway, seeing Dad in the condition he was in the last days before he passed was hard, but Charlotte's dream was encouraging for us that Dad was doing very well at this point. In the last few years, Dad would tell anyone who would listen that he was going to Heaven, even when he couldn't remember anything else. It is encouraging to know that this life isn't the end. I love my life here, but Heaven: I can only imagine!

One day we will get to see my Dad again. This encourages us as David says in Psalms 23 verse 4: "I may walk through a valley that is as dark as death. But I will not be afraid of any danger. This is because you are with me, Lord......" Also, I was listening to one of my favorite Bible teachers explain that the emotion that hinders us the most is fear. And what he says makes sense. Throughout the Bible many times we read that one of the characters was told not to fear. Such as when Jesus came walking on the water to his disciples, "But immediately Jesus said to them. 'Be brave! It is I. Do not be afraid.' ". Matthew 14:27. As we think back on our lives, I know this is true in my life, the times that we had our most difficult struggles were in times we were afraid. Afraid of failure, maybe ridicule, the unknown, loss, you name it.

Jesus wants us to know He will not fail us in any circumstance. Jesus faced the same fears we do, even the fear of death. Remember the Garden of Gethsemane, when Jesus prayed, He prayed, 'Father, if it is possible, please save me from this time of great pain. But Father, I do not ask you to do what I want. Do what you want to do.' in Matthew 26:39. Even in the Lord's prayer he prayed, "We want the day when you rule everyone to come soon. We want everyone to obey you on earth, like everyone in heaven obeys you."

Matthew 6:10. This should be our desire also. We have no reason to fear when God is in control and will accomplish what He desires. He wants only the best for us.

FEBRUARY, 2023

Dad's final death certificate has arrived. We were able to settle all of Dad's things. There are still a couple of doctor bills that will be taken care of by his insurance. We haven't seen James but all of the financial and legal matters are settled. We have settled into the house and are getting things updated as we go.

Things at school are going along. Some adjustments have been made by me and the school to accommodate the workload. They have been so good to me. I continue to seek God's will for my life. I keep hearing from different preachers that the process is the most important part of our life's journey, not the destination. I am aware of that but I still want to be where God wants me to be.

I do miss Dad. Putting together this book has been therapeutic for me. I have shed many tears and still do at times. It is a comfort knowing that with God's help and design, we did all we could for Dad, and one day we will see him and never part again.

But for now, on to the next chapter of our lives...

Bibliography

Voskamp, Ann, *One Thousand Gifts: A Dare to Live Fully Right Where You Are.* Grand Rapids, Mich., Zondervan, 2010. ISBN 9780310321910

Groeschel, Craig, *Hope in the Dark,* Zondervan. 08/21/2018. ISBN-13: 9780310342953

Voskamp, Ann, *One Thousand Gifts: A Dare to Live Fully Right Where You Are.* Grand Rapids, Mich., Zondervan, 2010. ISBN 9780310321910

Allen, Jennie, *Get Out of Your Head: Stopping the Spiral of Toxic Thoughts.* Crown Publishing Group, 2020. ISBN 9781601429667

http://www.jennieallen.com/podcast

David Jeremiah–https://www.davidjeremiah.org/

www.ingramcontent.com/pod-product-compliance
Lightning Source LLC
Chambersburg PA
CBHW060144240125

20772CB00002B/2